Cláudia Regina Gomes de Araujo
Ann Mary Feitosa Rosas

The nursing consultation in gynaecological brachytherapy treatment

Cláudia Regina Gomes de Araujo
Ann Mary Feitosa Rosas

The nursing consultation in gynaecological brachytherapy treatment

Imprint

Any brand names and product names mentioned in this book are subject to trademark, brand or patent protection and are trademarks or registered trademarks of their respective holders. The use of brand names, product names, common names, trade names, product descriptions etc. even without a particular marking in this work is in no way to be construed to mean that such names may be regarded as unrestricted in respect of trademark and brand protection legislation and could thus be used by anyone.

Cover image: www.ingimage.com

This book is a translation from the original published under ISBN 978-620-2-03981-9.

Publisher:
Sciencia Scripts
is a trademark of
Dodo Books Indian Ocean Ltd. and OmniScriptum S.R.L publishing group

120 High Road, East Finchley, London, N2 9ED, United Kingdom
Str. Armeneasca 28/1, office 1, Chisinau MD-2012, Republic of Moldova, Europe
Managing Directors: Ieva Konstantinova, Victoria Ursu
info@omniscriptum.com

Printed at: see last page
ISBN: 978-620-3-53573-0

Catalogue

DEDICATION

My respects go to the clients who undergo gynecological brachytherapy and the nurses who care for them.

SPECIAL THANKS TO THE GUIDE, PROF^(A)DR ANN MARY ROSAS

Learning to teach and learning from you has changed the way I experience caring. Thank you very much for agreeing to accompany me in this study.

ACKNOWLEDGMENTS

To God, for everything.

To my Spirit Guides, for taking care of me here on Earth.

To my grandmother Isabel Rosa Gomes, for the good memories she left me.

To my mother, Marilene Gomes de Araujo, for being with me all the time.

Marly de Faria Gomes, the best aunt I know.

To my siblings Isabel Cristina, Silvia Fernanda, Ana Paula and Luiz Alexandre, to whom I can tell everything, a big kiss.

To my nephews Raphael, Gabriela, Pietro, Carlos Eduardo, Luiz Henrique, Alexandre and Yasmim, for the mess we make when we're together. Sophia, we're waiting for you!

To my brother-in-law Erondy, for his help with the computer and with life's documents, always ready to help everyone.

The Nursing Division of the Clementino Fraga Filho University Hospital, for releasing me to carry out activities related to the course, especially my immediate boss, Nurse Michele Oliveira, for making it possible for me to take time off to study with such commitment.

To the Nursing Team at the Barretos Cancer Hospital, for their professional and affectionate welcome. Thank you, Talita, Sabrina, Roberto, Ana Paula, Brenda and Sandra. I will always remember you.

To the Research Ethics Committee of the Barretos Cancer Hospital, for understanding my study so well and treating me as if I were from the institution, especially to the secretaries Ricardo, Daniela and Bruna, for their attention.

The postgraduate secretariat of the Anna Nery School of Nursing, in the person of Jorge Anselmo and Sonia, for their help with administrative issues.

The secretariat of the Study Center of the Hospital Escola Sao Francisco de Assis, in the person of Rose and Ana Carla, for their dedication and availability to all of us students.

To the teachers and colleagues of the subjects taken during the course, thank you very much for everything I learned from you.

To the members of the examining board, Prof^a Dr$^{(a)}$Benedita Rodrigues, Prof^1 Dr$^{(a)}$Ligia Viana, Prof^s Dr$^{(a)}$ Terezinha Silva, Prof$^{(3)}$Dr$^{(3)}$Neiva Santos, Prof^s Dr$^{(a)}$ Laisa Alcantara and Prof^s Dr$^{(a)}$ Maria Helena Souza, for their contributions during the construction of the study, especially Profª Bend, for her affection.

My classmate Alexandra, for her companionship and help during the course.

To my colleagues Claudia and Renata, for their camaraderie and for sharing so much teaching and learning. We've got a lot of work ahead of us, girls!

My most recent mentor, Maria Amalia, who came to help me.

To my teammates, for filling in for me so well while I carried out the study. Thank you, Suze, Maria de Fatima, Therezinha, Valdecy, Adriana and Maria Fatima. Thank you for your strength!

To my friend and coworker Renata Henze, for the acupuncture sessions and for listening to me when I found everything so difficult.

To everyone who helped me with the computer, especially my brother Xandre and my work partner Fatima. Thanks Shock, thanks Fafa!

To everyone I met along the way who helped me resolve the various issues related to the course. Thank you so much! I certainly couldn't have done it alone.

SUMMARY

TEACHING AND LEARNING IN THE NURSING CONSULTATION BETWEEN CLIENTS AND NURSES IN GYNECOLOGICAL BRACHYTHERAPY TREATMENT: A PHENOMENOLOGICAL APPROACH

My interest in this study arose from my work as a nurse in the radiotherapy department of a general, public, university hospital in the city of Rio de Janeiro (RJ). Its theme is learning to teach and learning to think about the experiences of clients and nurses in the nursing consultation for gynecological brachytherapy treatment. This is a qualitative, descriptive and exploratory study based on Phenomenology. The **object of** the study was the meaning of teaching and learning in the nursing consultation during gynecological brachytherapy treatment, according to the expectations of clients and nurses. The **objectives** were to identify the expectations of clients and nurses in teaching and learning in the nursing consultation in gynecological brachytherapy treatment and to discuss the links between the intentions expressed by nurses and clients about teaching and learning in the nursing consultation in gynecological brachytherapy treatment. The study **settings** were the Radiotherapy Department of the Clementino Fraga Filho University Hospital, Federal University of Rio de Janeiro, and the Radiotherapy Department of the Barretos Cancer Hospital, Pio XII Foundation. **Methodology:** The subjects were thirteen female clients over the age of eighteen undergoing gynecological brachytherapy and six nurses working in the aforementioned settings. Authorizations were granted by the Research Ethics Committees of these institutions under numbers 127/11 and 551/2011, respectively. The statements were analyzed in the light of Alfred Schutz's Sociological Phenomenology. Clients and nurses expressed their expectations about teaching and learning in the nursing consultation during gynecological brachytherapy treatment. **Results:** The following concrete categories of what was experienced emerged from the clients' statements: *Seeking Grientagoes, Experiencing Fear and Overcoming Pain.* Thus, it can be said that the clients' lived experience is that of people who need guidance, are afraid of the disease and the treatment and experience physical and emotional pain caused by the diagnosis and the procedures. The following concrete categories of what was experienced emerged from the nurses' statements: *Attending to the Singularity of Subjects in Treatment and Valuing Technical Care.* Thus, it can be said that the type lived by the nurses interviewed is that of professionals with the sensitivity to adapt individual care to technology. **Final considerations:** The study revealed a clientele that looks to nurses as a reference point when seeking guidance on how to deal with treatment. The teaching and learning that emerges in the nursing consultation for clients undergoing gynaecological brachytherapy helps nurses to understand that each client has a different level of understanding and that it is important to personalize this teaching in order to care for the other, so that every client has quality of life during treatment. Thus, I reiterate the value of learning to teach and learning to think about the experiences between clients and nurses in the nursing consultation for gynecological brachytherapy treatment.

Keywords: role of the nursing professional, nursing care, radiotherapy, brachytherapy, nursing education

SUMMARY

1. INITIAL CONSIDERATIONS

This chapter deals with the author's background, contextualization of the object of study, guiding question, objectives, justification and contribution.

INITIAL CONSIDERATIONS

The first memory that comes to mind when I reflect on the study is of the clients in the radiotherapy ward, totally absorbed in the procedures, looking for the nurse, as if they couldn't bear our absence. Without a doubt, I think it's impossible to do nursing without the empathy needed to experience the technical and scientific issues of the life world of this profession of being a nurse.

Professional experience shows that care must go beyond technology, including touch and the exchange of glances, which cannot be described in words. Thus, caring for clients with cancer, a disease that carries with it the stigma of approaching death and a life that is dubious in relation to health standards, requires sensitivity and effective knowledge of their basic human needs.

In the case of women with uterine cancer, a disease that violates the intimacy of the human being, feelings of embarrassment, denial and doubt can arise. With the diagnosis of the disease, it is common for clients to evaluate their position in life and their social network, such as family, community and their own being in the world of life. While practicing care, I was able to see the closeness that is established between clients and the nursing team, due to the very nature of this care, which takes place throughout the client's treatment process. All of this provides an opportunity for exchange, in terms of teaching and learning, for both the caregiver and the one being cared for.

The personal experience of care to which I refer takes place in the Radiotherapy Service of a general, public, university hospital in the city of Rio de Janeiro (RJ), where I work as a nurse. This service was inaugurated in 2002 through the

of the Expande Project, developed by the Brazilian Ministry of Health (MS), in partnership with the Jose Alencar Gomes da Silva National Cancer Institute (INCA).

As a requirement for working in an oncology sector, the Ministry of Health recommends that nurses working in these sectors should be specialists, or at least one member of the team should be. The other nurses should receive training in specialized institutions, until it is possible to take the course in question, in accordance with the rules described in Ordinance GM/MS nº 3.535, of 1998, of the Expande Project (BRASIL, MS, 2011).

So, in order to meet the requirements of the Ministry of Health, I took the Oncology Nursing Specialization course at INCA in 2002. This course resulted in a monograph on nursing consultations with tracheostomized clients. With this, it was possible to systematize nursing care for clients with head and neck cancer, in the sector in which I work, including basing care for clients with tracheostomies (TQT), justifying the attention that nurses give to them (TQT) during treatment (ARAUJO, 2002).

The specialty pushed me to continue my studies. In 2007, I completed my Master's degree at the Anna Nery School of Nursing (EEAN) at the Federal University of Rio de Janeiro (UFRJ). The dissertation was developed through the Nursing Education and Health Research Center (NUPESENF), of the Nursing Methodology Department, with the title "The meaning of the nursing consultation in the radiotherapy sector of the Clementino Fraga Filho University Hospital, in the approach of clients and caregivers" (ARAUJO, 2007).

The results of this dissertation, which used Alfred Schutz's Sociological Phenomenology as its theoretical-methodological framework, helped us to understand how and why clients and caregivers recognize the importance of the nursing consultation in the sector in question. Through what was said by the subjects of the study, the reasons why they attend the first meeting with the nurse, return for subsequent nursing appointments and carry out the prescribed nursing care were understood.

These motivations come from their basic needs, which in turn originate from their life history, their lived experience, how they are experiencing the reality of their illness and treatment. According to their testimonies, after going through the nursing consultation, the clients became interested in learning how to practice self-care, and their relatives became interested in learning how to look after them. Both clients and caregivers were unaware of the nursing consultation until they attended it. What we found afterwards was that people were satisfied and confident with the guidance and care provided. We also concluded that the process of teaching and learning that takes place in the nursing consultation (NC) gives rise to the nurse's motivation to care.

It was clear that the implementation of the nursing consultation in the Radiotherapy Service has benefited clients and their caregivers, enabling quality of life during treatment. This experience has revealed a clientele that looks to nurses as a reference point when seeking guidance on how to deal with treatment.

In fact, the care provided through EC is one of the many activities that nurses carry out in the radiotherapy service described in this study. Initially, the role of the nursing team raised doubts among the other members of the multidisciplinary team, who were unaware of their role and questioned the reason for the presence of nurses and nursing technicians in the sector.

Therefore, in parallel with the implementation of our work project, stimulating activities were carried out to raise awareness among the Radiotherapy Service team, in order to clarify aspects related to our activities. I have to say that the space gained by the nursing team since then has been significant, although I recognize that we can go further. Let me make it clear that the multi-professional team, apart from the nursing team, is made up of doctors, physicists, nutritionists, social workers, psychologists, X-ray technicians, secretaries and cleaners.

Radiotherapy care, according to the service's routine, involves specific nursing activities, such as nebulization, administration of medication, referrals to the various sectors, accompaniment to exams and medical procedures, dressings, care of the tracheostomy and all the material used in the sector.

Nurses are responsible for planning, coordinating and providing nursing care to the sector's clients, while highly complex care and nursing consultations are their own activities and cannot be delegated. Teaching, research and extension activities are also the exclusive responsibility of the nurse, as is the coordination of the entire operation of the outpatient department, including the provision of materials for the service.

Nursing technicians are responsible for providing comprehensive care to clients in the sector, under the supervision of the nurse, in activities such as checking vital signs, helping to position the client on the treatment table, assisting with the client's physical examination, performing simple dressings, administering medication, among others.

Hospitalized clients are the responsibility of the nurse and their team during their stay in the Radiotherapy Department, in order to guarantee continuity of care. As for outpatients, they are accompanied by this team at all times and receive nursing care whenever necessary.

Therefore, I identify that nurses and their team act as a link between clients, caregivers and the multidisciplinary team, being present at all stages of radiotherapy treatment. Therefore, they are also involved in the educational process for clients and their families, by providing guidance. The teaching and learning that takes place at this time helps us to understand that each client has different levels of understanding and that it is important to personalize this teaching in order to care for the other.

It is a fact that each client is unique, since, for Schutz (1979, 2012), every human being is unique, possessing their own individuality. And each individual, in the process of becoming ill, is learning to position themselves in the world of life, going through moments that are not always easy to deal with. That said, nurses are the professionals with the skills to identify their complaints and needs, learning how each of their clients acts, without departing from technical-scientific knowledge and humanizing their actions and reactions.

Continuing the implementation of the aforementioned care model, with the introduction of gynecological brachytherapy, the role of nursing intensified in the service. This team is responsible for guiding clients and participating with the multidisciplinary team in all the steps of the procedure, as well as taking care of the material used in the technique. The nurse is also responsible for organizing the department and providing the necessary infrastructure for the treatment to take place.

The learning acquired during my master's degree changed my intentional approach to care and encouraged me to reflect on the ways of practicing nursing, through contact with the various areas of this profession's body of knowledge.

As a result of these reflections and the results of the dissertation, two articles were published. The first, in the Revista de Enfermagem da UERJ, focused on the nursing consultation for clients and their caregivers in the radiotherapy sector of a university hospital (ARAUJO and ROSAS, 2008). The second, in the Revista Brasileira de Cancerologia, on the role of the nursing team in the radiotherapy sector and their contribution to the multidisciplinary team (ARAUJO and ROSAS, 2008).

The impact of this second publication resulted in an invitation to present this work at a radiotherapy event at an institution in Barretos (SP). With its advanced technology, this hospital encouraged me to develop a study describing the experiences of clients and nurses in teaching and learning from the nursing consultation in gynecological brachytherapy treatment.

And, as a motivation for this study, just as it was possible to structure nursing care for clients undergoing external radiotherapy in the sector where I work, I now aim to direct this study towards clients undergoing internal radiotherapy, gynecological brachytherapy. The previous reflections have also led to the desire to reformulate the care model that exists in the service, in which it would be possible to listen to the clients, give voice to their needs and plan the care, adapting it to these needs. Obviously, without forgetting the reality of the institution, taking into account its resources, philosophy, goals, mission and objectives.

It is important to emphasize that it is not a question of comparing the care provided by the nurses in the two institutions, but of adding knowledge to the foundation of care. The teaching and learning between clients and nurses in the nursing consultation has the singularity of experiences and diverse cultures. I believe that, although these clients have a common clinical diagnosis, the uniqueness of each one's speech will help to recreate new forms of nursing care.

That said, it was decided that there would be two sites for this study: the first was the Radiotherapy Department of a general, public, university hospital in Rio de Janeiro, as already mentioned. This institution serves clients of the Unified Health System (SUS) and is dedicated to teaching, research, assistance and extension. It is the Clementino Fraga Filho University Hospital (HUCFF), of the Federal University of Rio de Janeiro (UFRJ). The second site is the Radiotherapy Department of a philanthropic hospital, maintained by a Foundation, which also serves clients via SUS. This institution specializes in oncology and has assistance, prevention, teaching, research and extension programs in cancer treatment. It is located in Barretos (SP). It is the Barretos Cancer Hospital of the Pio XII Foundation.

Regarding the models of care at both institutions, the following realities are apparent: the Barretos institution, for logistical reasons, carries out the nursing consultation for clients undergoing brachytherapy (BQT) at the time they are oriented for teletherapy, which is the stage prior to the aforementioned treatment (BQT). And throughout the treatment, the clients are monitored by the nurses. As for the institution in Rio de Janeiro, there is a desire to reformulate the existing consultation model, giving the clients a voice.

In this way, the two scenarios in this study can go through a process of reconstructing the nursing consultation for the type of client referred to, if they so wish. I believe that the foundation of nursing care, combined with the questioning of clients about how they are experiencing treatment and the questioning of nurses about how they reflect on care, will provide instruments for proposing a model that suits the clients' needs.

And with this reflection, I reaffirm my interest in developing a study in which part of the knowledge of the reality of a general, public and university hospital is combined with part of the knowledge of the reality of a hospital specialized in oncology, philanthropic, focused on teaching and research. The partnership formed with the nurses at the Barretos Cancer Hospital was essential for achieving this goal, as well as being constructive.

Both institutions have four fundamental lines of cancer treatment: surgery, chemotherapy, radiotherapy and bone marrow transplantation. The focus of the study was gynecological brachytherapy, known as contact radiotherapy.

Radiotherapy can be defined as a method capable of destroying tumour cells using beams of ionizing radiation. A pre-calculated dose of radiation is applied, over a given period of time, to a volume of tissue that encompasses the tumor, with the aim of eradicating all tumor cells, with as little damage as possible to the surrounding normal cells, at the expense of which the irradiated area will regenerate. It can be used at any stage of cancer treatment, for therapeutic or palliative purposes (BRASIL, MS, INCA, 2002a, 2012).

When used for therapeutic purposes, the aim is to try to cure or control the disease. When used for palliative purposes, the aim is to control symptoms and promote comfort by decompressing structures. This decompression of structures acts to relieve pain, improve dyspnea, improve movement, free the lumen of an organ or stop bleeding, providing quality of life for the client (AYOUB et al, 2000; BRASIL, MS, INCA, 2012).

It is an effective treatment because it destroys tumor cells. Irradiation can be applied at a distance (teletherapy) or directly to the tumor, without reaching adjacent structures (brachytherapy). In brachytherapy, seeds or applicators are introduced into a body cavity, any affected tissue or channel. The radioactive source is therefore in physical contact with the client. The dose of radiation applied close to the source is very high and decreases as you move away from it. This spares the tissues far from the source (BRASIL, MS, INCA, 2002a; UICC, 2006; BRASIL, MS, INCA, 2012).

The apparatus used in the Radiotherapy Department at HUCFF/UFRJ for teletherapy is a linear accelerator. For gynecological brachytherapy, an Iridium source[192] and intravaginal applicators are used. It is therefore an invasive procedure, performed under anesthesia (sedation). The aim of this treatment is to control or cure cervical cancer, endometrium and vagina.

Gynecological brachytherapy began at the RJ hospital in January 2007. With its implementation, a nursing consultation (NC) was instituted for clients undergoing the procedure. There is usually a nursing consultation at the beginning and another at the end of the treatment, which on average lasts a month.

It was found that clients who receive a nursing consultation before treatment are able to cope with it more calmly. In fact, on several occasions, this peace of mind contributed to a reduction in anesthesia time, a fact observed in the day-to-day care. Therefore, the consultations reduce anxiety and help clients understand what brachytherapy is.

As explained above, the practice of caring made it possible to understand what happened to the clients before and after the nursing consultation for the modality in question was instituted. The evidence of nursing care revealed that an informed and collaborative client copes better with treatment and optimizes procedure time. I agree with Gates & Fink et al (2009) when they say that information is a powerful tool.

I understand that the moment of the nursing consultation consists of an exchange of experiences and knowledge, between the one who consults and the one who is consulted. It's an activity that has been developing more and more in health units, requiring improvement in its technique. It's not uncommon for clients to complain about the lack of guidance when they don't go to the nurse for a consultation. Likewise, it's not uncommon for nurses to marvel at the resolving power of a properly conducted consultation.

When nurses teach their clients, they are helping them to reproduce the care they received during the nursing consultation in their daily lives. And when the clients come back and report the results of the nursing consultation, they realize that it was possible to learn from them about their needs. In other words, nurses learn from their clients how they perceive their health situation and how they experience self-care issues.

The following important statement from a client, found in the work by Figueiredo et al (2009, p. 453), corroborates the importance of this type of exchange:

"As I waited for my treatment in the radiotherapy waiting room, I watched those clients who were there, without any guidance, lacking any moral, spiritual, physical assistance or anything else you can imagine. I saw those people having their radiotherapy and then going off to the countryside to start the same life, not knowing about the treatment, not knowing what they were doing to their bodies, learning from each other. I told the doctor about my concerns and he asked me what I would suggest and I said: that there should be a team with a nurse, a social worker and a psychologist, to support these people, who had come from the countryside and were spitting on the floor, not knowing what they were going to do with their lives".

It is clear from this report how important the nurse's guidance is for clients, and the statement is an example of what should be avoided. And looking at the procedure in question (gynecological brachytherapy), the author of this study couldn't think otherwise.

Thus, understanding the importance of the interaction between those involved in the treatment in question, the **question guiding** the study is: how do clients and nurses experience the teaching and learning that nursing consultations provide in gynecological brachytherapy treatment?

The **object of** the study is the meaning of teaching and learning in the nursing consultation in the treatment of gynecological brachytherapy in the expectation of clients and nurses.

The **objectives** were to identify the expectations of clients and nurses in teaching and learning in the nursing consultation in gynecological brachytherapy treatment and to discuss the links between the intentions expressed by nurses and clients about teaching and learning in the nursing consultation in gynecological brachytherapy treatment.

I believe that the educational process that takes place during nursing consultations enlightens both clients and nurses, helping clients to optimize their self-care and nurses to plan their care.

The aim is to find out what clients expect from EC and what it means for nurses to provide care through these nursing consultations. In this way, it will be possible for the HUCFF Radiotherapy Service to update the current nursing care model for these clients, adapting care to their needs.

To support the thesis, a bibliographic search was carried out in the Virtual Health Library, consulting the LILACS, BDENF, MEDLINE and IBECS databases, without a time cut-off and with selection in Portuguese, English and Spanish. I used the following descriptors: Role of the Nursing Professional, Nursing Care, Radiotherapy, Brachytherapy and Nursing Education.

I identified studies on nursing care in oncology, focusing on the importance of the nurse's role in this type of care and the coping strategies adopted by clients during the proposed treatment.

Among these, Muniz, Zago and Schwartz (2009) state that each person with cancer is a survivor of treatment, with unique needs based on the extent of the disease. And these people establish partnerships (weave webs) around them in order to live with the reality of having the pathology in question. Thus, according to Machado and Sawada (2008), nursing plays an important role in controlling the effects and consequences of treatment as a whole, and its responsibility goes beyond technical care.

The study by Rosa and Sales (2008) on the experience of women undergoing gynecological brachytherapy stood out among those visited in the literature, as it described the routine that the client goes through during the treatment process, providing information about her universe. Considering this universe, Feijo, Schwartz, Jardim, Linck, Zillmer and Lange (2009), apprdached nursing care in oncology, focusing on the role of the family for the client, which translates into a foundation for them.

I would like to highlight the existence of studies on the importance of nurses specializing in oncology in the radiotherapy sector. This emphasizes the need for this professional to be increasingly trained, as Diegues and Pires pointed out in 1997.

I also identified studies that highlighted the value of educational activities in nursing consultations. Two of these were on educational practice in nursing consultations, with a focus on children's learning (Santana, 2002) and on communicative action and its contribution to nursing consultations (Machado, Leitao and Holanda, 2005).

In view of the above, this thesis **is justified** by the importance of listening to clients and nurses about their educational needs, with the aim of directing nursing actions towards the reasons that bring them to the nursing consultation. Teaching and learning with clients and nurses is useful when it comes to substantiating the scientificity of the care provided. As the uniqueness of the subjects of this study is not to be found in books, I went in search of it in order to get to know them. By getting to know each client and nurse, I got to know their singularities. This led to the knowledge of the interviewees' typicality. And since each statement was unique, I was able to learn from each person interviewed.

The importance of recording a model of care leads us to reflect on the Systematization of

Nursing Care (SNC), instituted by the Ministry of Health to meet the needs of health care for human groups (BRASIL, MS, 2009). In this sense, with the continuous process of teaching and learning in the nursing consultation, the nurses will be able to reconstruct their care model in the Radiotherapy Service, becoming a reference for other institutions, including the creation of didactic material for the consultation (explanatory leaflet).

When I chose two reference institutions for uterine cancer treatment, I made sure that the therapy offered was similar, with types of clientele that had common facts, such as clinical diagnosis, the fact that they were women and the experience of treatment. The existing nuances (such as lifestyle and access to the health system) are typical of the reality of each location, and do not interfere with the search for answers. As the clinical diagnosis of the clients interviewed is the same, it was possible, at the end of this thesis, to see what is in common between these clients and the nurses, in the two institutions, when teaching and learning in the nursing consultation for the client undergoing gynecological brachytherapy.

This apprehension of meaning came about through knowledge of the lived experience and uniqueness of each person interviewed, both client and nurse, and what teaching and learning mean to them, respectively. Subsequently, the lived type of client and the lived type of nurse who experience teaching and learning in the nursing consultation emerged; lived type (Schutz, 1979, 2012) being understood as the description of how the subject experiences a given biographical situation.

I also believe in the possibility of reflecting on the reality of two similar but different universes, with their own culture and resources. And in this way, I can learn to teach and learn from the subjects of this study, nurses and clients of the institutions mentioned.

The relevance of the study lies in the fact that cancer is a reality in people's lives that needs to be faced. And the more knowledge available to those who have to look after their clients, the better they will be able to respond to the need to cope.

The role of nursing in the field of oncology has kept pace with technological and scientific development, and the subject is being explored in our environment. In order to meet this new type of demand, there are specialization courses in oncology nursing in Brazil and the articulation of oncology nursing teaching in undergraduate nursing courses is already taking place.

Popim and Boemer (2005) warn of the need to increase the number of qualified oncology professionals, pointing out that this specialty requires both technical and scientific skills and interpersonal skills. And in the case of radiotherapy, it is a specialty within another, which is oncology.

Another relevant fact is that the number of cases of uterine cancer in Brazil and worldwide is significant, according to estimates by the Ministry of Health. Statistics show that more than 30,000 new cases of the disease have emerged in recent years. According to the Ministry of Health, in 2008 there were 4,812 deaths caused by the disease. As these numbers continue to rise, they reiterate the importance of preventing the disease in the country (BRASIL, MS, INCA, 2008, 2012).

When you study the effects of cancer on the human body, you come to the conclusion that it is a huge disease. However, there are two advantages in the fight against it: the possibility of prevention and the ability to obtain an early diagnosis. To this end, education is essential in the fight against the disease. Therefore, every effort will be wasted when it comes to providing information in order to prevent, diagnose and treat the disease. It is therefore clear to see the value of the teaching-learning process and the positive impact it can have on people's lives, which can even change the way they live with the fact that they are ill.

The study's **contribution** is aimed at teaching those who wish to delve deeper into the subject, with a view to reaching undergraduate students who are starting out in the profession, postgraduate students who are specializing, teachers and care professionals interested in working in the area. This exchange can also take place between institutions providing care, teaching, research and extension, focused on oncology, through study groups.

When we share knowledge, we are propagating the foundations of nursing care , which encourages reflection on the profession's body of knowledge. In this way, we will be able to provide input for other research that may emerge, not only from health and education professionals, but also from the technology sector.

This is a product of the Nursing Education and Health Research Center (NUPESENF) of the Methodology Department of the Anna Nery Nursing School (EEAN) of the Federal University of Rio de Janeiro (UFRJ). The NUPESENF has been disseminating studies in the area of nursing education and health, helping to consolidate the knowledge of this profession (VIANA, SANTOS, VALENTE, ROSAS, SANTOS & SILVA, 2009). Therefore, the publication of the results found here, in partnership with NUPESENF, is the author's intention, in order to accompany the growth that the group has achieved today.

This thesis changed the author's view of care and contributed to the reconstruction of the care model at the HUCFF Radiotherapy Service. Updating the text of the explanatory leaflet for clients and updating the service's protocols were the first fruits of this work. The organization of other documents from the sector in question and the carrying out of scientific activities for future generations of nurses at the Service will also be legacies of this study. By disseminating the nurse's way of caring in the HUCFF radiotherapy department, I hope to provide readers with what I have learned and taught along this journey.

This study is therefore aimed at clients facing gynecological brachytherapy treatment and the nurses who care for them, highlighting the value of partnership between human beings.

2. UTERINE AND VAGINAL CANCER

This chapter covers concepts relating to uterine and vaginal cancer and some of the ways of preventing it.

UTERINE AND VAGINAL CANCER

This chapter is designed to provide a more detailed understanding of the universe of the client who undergoes gynecological brachytherapy. The technical information presented here was drawn from the literature of the Instituto Nacional de Cancer Tc3ë Alencar Gomes da Silva (BRASIL, MS, INCA, 2008, 2012), an organ of the Ministry of Health (MS), which focuses on oncology research and care in the country, and is a specialized institution and a reference on the subject.

The Ministry of Health, through INCA and other institutions prepared for this, has been updating and guaranteeing comprehensive care for clients with cancer in Brazil, establishing a classification of the centers that provide oncological care. Thus, the High Complexity Oncology Centers (CACONs) were created, which are public or philanthropic hospital units that offer the four main lines of treatment for cancer: surgery, chemotherapy, radiotherapy and bone marrow transplantation (BRASIL, MS, 2011).

In 1998, Ministerial Order 3.535 was published by the Ministry of Health, which regulates the treatment of malignant neoplasms, establishing a public health policy against this pathology and proposing measures for the prevention, early detection and diagnosis of the disease. The result of this work is reported annually, with the publication of two reports: Estimated Cancer in Brazil and Cancer Incidence and Mortality in Brazil, by the MS (BRASIL, MS, 2011).

The most common types of uterine cancer are divided into two:

2.1 CERVICAL CANCER

Cancer (CA) is a chronic degenerative disease in which the disordered growth of cells invades tissues and organs and can spread throughout the body. It evolves with lesions that take the form of an expansive solid tumor and/or infiltrate body structures (BRASIL, MS, INCA, 2008, 2012).

Cervical tumors develop from changes in the cervix, a structure located deep inside the vagina. It can arise from repeated infections with the human papillomavirus (HPV). This virus plays an important role in the development of cervical cancer, as it causes precursor lesions to tumors in the uterine epithelium and is present in more than 90% of cervical cancer cases (BRASIL, MS, INCA, 2012).

Among the main causal factors are the early onset of sexual activity, sexual promiscuity, family history, smoking and obesity. Prevention is easy. The main weapons against the disease are the use of condoms and regular preventive gynecological examinations. It is also important to avoid sexual contact with multiple partners (BRASIL, MS, INCA, 2012).

Exploring the subject in the media has helped in the fight against cancer in general, by providing the population with educational content. The use of campaigns and leaflets is useful in breaking down taboos, especially when talking about sex with young people.

Preventive examinations (Pap smears) are important for detecting precursor lesions to tumors. According to INCA (2012), if the disease is diagnosed at an early stage, a 100% cure rate is possible. This is relevant, since the disease can be silent in its early stages. Bleeding, vaginal discharge and abdominal pain are signs that appear as the disease progresses, when the woman could already be being treated. Therefore, time is of the essence when it comes to controlling and curing any type of cancer.

According to Gates and Fink et al (2009), cervical cancer is characterized by a slow pre-invasive and pre-malignant state. These lesions can regress, persist or become invasive. It can take up to seven years for early changes to progress to an invasive tumor. This is why the MoH says it is so important to detect the disease early on.

The gynecological preventive exam should be carried out according to certain criteria: it is recommended that the woman is not menstruating and that she is asked not to have sexual intercourse or use vaginal cream two days before the exam. These measures are in place so that the result is obtained more reliably. The test should be repeated according to the woman's general condition and the doctor's request.

And, most importantly, the client should undergo the preventive examination, **get** the result and take it to her doctor to continue her CA prevention/treatment program. These recommendations apply to all women, especially those who are of childbearing age and have an active sex life. Pregnant women can also undergo gynecological preventive examinations (BRASIL, MS, INCA, 2012).

Still thinking about prevention, one cannot fail to mention how fundamental the use of condoms is, whether male or female. The male condom is cheaper and easier to use and is distributed in health centers. The female condom was registered in Brazil in 1997 with the National Health Surveillance Agency (ANVISA). Although it has been available on the Brazilian market since December of that year, it is little known, more difficult to use and poorly supplied in health services (BRASIL, MS, INCA, 2012).

Another tool that can be used to prevent uterine cancer is the HPV vaccine. However, according to the Ministry of Health (2012), it is still under study and does not protect against all subtypes of the virus, and its administration is still restricted to private institutions.

Gynecological cancers are staged according to the guidelines established by the International Federation of Gynecology and Obstetrics (FIGO), with treatment designated according to the size, type of tumor, general condition of the client and location of the tumor (GATES & FINK et al, 2009). Still referring to the authors, the staging of cervical cancer follows:

Stage I - Confined to the cdrvix

Stage IA1 - Stromal invasion < 3mm deep and < 7mm wide

Stage IA2 - Stromal invasion > 3 mm to 5 mm deep and < 7 mm wide

Stage IBi - Stromal invasion > 5 mm deep or > 7 mm wide and clinical lesions < 4 cm

Stage IB2 - Clinical lesions > 4 cm

Stage II - Extension beyond the cdrvix and/or upper two tergos of the vagina

Stage IIA - No parametrial involvement

Stage IIB - Parametrial involvement

Stage III - Extension to the lower end of the vagina

Stage IIIA - No extension to the lateral wall of the pelvis

Stage IIIB - Extension to the lateral wall of the pelvis and/or hydronephrosis

Stage IV - Extension aldm of the small pelvis

Stage IVA - Involvement of adjacent organs (bladder, rectum)

Stage IVB - Distant metastases

2.2 ENDOMETRIAL CANCER

It often occurs in post-menopausal women aged between 55 and 70. It is rarer under the age of 40. Its detection is common through cervical cancer screening, just as it is with vaginal cancer. The risk factors for this type of tumor are early onset of menstruation, menopause, obesity, nulliparity, diabetes and hypertension (MOHALLEM & RODRIGUES et al, 2007).

Staging of endometrial cancer (GATES & FINK et al, 2009):

Stage I - Confined to the endometrium

Est. IA - Limited to the endometrium

Stage IB - Invades < half of the myometrium

IC stage - Invades > half of the myometrium

Est. II - The edrvice is extended

Stage IIA - Involves endocervical glands

Stage IIB - Invades cervical stroma

Stage III - Involves adjacent structures

Stage IIIA - Invades uterine serosa, appendages, or positive peritoneal cytology

Stage IIIB - Vaginal extension

Stage IIIC - Metastases to pelvic or para-aortic lymph nodes

2.3 VAGINAL CANCER

It has a rare incidence and can be located in any part of the organ, but the most common location is in the upper tergium of the posterior part (closest to the cervix). It occurs in all age groups and most tumors are secondary to disease in adjacent regions. Only in approximately 15 to 20% of cases do tumors start in the vagina (MOHALLEM & RODRIGUES et al, 2007).

Staging (BRASIL, MS, INCA, 2012):

Stage 0 - Intraepithelial invasion

Stage I - Limited to the vaginal wall

Stage II - Extends to sub-vaginal tissue

Stage III - Extends to the pelvic wall

Stage IV - Extends to one side of the bladder or compromises the bladder mucosa

Stage IV A - Involvement of adjacent organs

Section B - Involvement of remote bodies

In all the above-mentioned types of tumor, the signs may be as follows, and women should be aware of them:

- Presence of vaginal fluid that is different from the woman's normal patterns (that's why it's important to know about it), dark in color, modified and with a foul odor.

- Bleeding after sex.

- Pain during and after sex.

- Irregular vaginal bleeding.

- Pain in the abdominal, pelvic and/or lumbar region.

In view of the above, the importance of the work of nurses and their teams is clear, as they act both in prevention programs and in the treatment of the disease.

3. GYNECOLOGICAL BRACHYTHERAPY PROCEDURE ROUTINE IN THE STUDY SECTORS

This chapter describes the routines of the gynecological brachytherapy procedure at the hospitals in Rio de Janeiro and Barretos.

BRACHYTHERAPY ROUTINE IN THE STUDY SETTINGS

In brachytherapy (contact radiotherapy), the radiation is applied directly to the tumor using intracavitary applicators, implants with needles or molds. Its advantage is that it better protects the structures adjacent to the tumor, because the energy is centralized in the tumor and can even be greater than the energy used in teletherapy (external radiation). It is an invasive procedure and is always performed after teletherapy in order to complement the treatment (BRASIL, MS, INCA, 2009).

In the radiotherapy department at HUCFF, an Iridium[192] source is used for brachytherapy. This ionizing radiation is stored in a safe and released via computer control. Currently, only gynecological brachytherapy is being performed, for the treatment of uterine and vaginal tumors.

Below, we explain how gynecological brachytherapy is carried out at the hospital. To this end, the roles of the professionals involved in the treatment were highlighted and the flow of clients in the sector was described. The steps of the procedure were also described and the competencies of the nursing team were specified. It should be noted that gynecological brachytherapy in this sector is an activity that requires the participation of professionals from various areas, in an interdisciplinary way in which each one must know their role and act when necessary to assist the client.

The professionals involved in the procedure and their respective roles are:

Nurse: looks after the client and manages the running of the room, providing the infrastructure for the treatment to take place. Their competence will be described in more detail below.

Nursing technician: assists the nurse in all tasks related to treatment.

Radiotherapist: prescribes the brachytherapy dose, inserts and removes the applicators.

Anesthetist: responsible for providing the client with the necessary analgesia, as this is a painful and invasive procedure.

Physicist: calculates the distribution of the radiation dose through the tissues and operates the apparatus used in the treatment.

Radiotherapy technician: performs X-rays on the client to confirm proper positioning of the applicator.

Cleaning staff: responsible for cleaning the room after each procedure.

The flow of clients who are to undergo brachytherapy is as follows:

- The client is assessed by the radiotherapist, after having undergone teletherapy, to confirm the need for brachytherapy.

- If the need is confirmed, the brachytherapy will be scheduled at the ward office. After this appointment, the client receives guidance from the nurse about the procedure during the consultation.

- The client must come to the department for the treatment, according to the appointment made at the secretariat. In the case of gynecological brachytherapy, the treatment is carried out in four sessions, one week apart, taking an average of one month to complete.

- At the end of the treatment, the client makes a final appointment with the radiotherapy doctor for a review.

- The client returns to her original doctor, either the oncologist or the gynecologist who referred her for radiotherapy.

Procedure steps:

- The client is welcomed into the ward, must be fasting and accompanied by a family member or friend. This should be checked by the nursing staff.

- The nurse and/or nursing technician positions the client on the treatment table, leaving her in the gynecological position.

- The X-ray technician confirms the client's position on the table for the X-ray.

- The client is anesthetized by the anesthesiologist, while the radiotherapist gets ready for the procedure.

- A bladder catheter is placed in the client, and the balloon of the catheter is filled with iodine-based contrast solution so that the bladder can be visualized through the X-ray. The need to identify the bladder on the X-ray is imperative so that, when the physicist calculates and distributes the radiation dose to the tissues, the noble structures that are most sensitive to radiation are protected and given smaller amounts when the calculation is made. In the case of gynecological brachytherapy, the most sensitive structures are the bladder, the sigmoid curve and the rectum, which is why the bladder needs to be identified on the X-ray. The X-ray is also important because it helps to visualize the correct positioning of the applicator (UICC, 2006; PELLIZZON et al, 2008).

- Placement of the vaginal speculum and applicator by the radiotherapist. The tray with all the material used is previously arranged by the nurse, who assists the doctor when inserting the applicator.

- The physicist connects the applicator to the device containing the Iridium source, using a temporary cable, just for radiography.

- The RxT technician performs the X-ray.

- Using the X-ray image, the physicist calculates the dose.

- The definitive energy transmitter cables are laid by the physicist.

- The treatment begins. During the treatment, the client remains alone in the room, but is observed through a screen. In the event of complications, the application can be interrupted at any time. To avoid this, it is useful to check the client's general condition before she leaves the room.

- After treatment, the applicator and bladder catheter are removed by the radiotherapist. The nurse helps at this point and can remove the applicator, **provided they are trained** to do so.

- The client is removed from the table by the nurse and/or nursing technician. The nurse should assess the client's general condition, making sure she is recovering, before releasing her. The necessary instructions can also be given when the client is released.

- Release the client after she has eaten, and always accompanied.

- The instruments used are removed from the room and taken for disinfection.

- The cleaning lady cleans the room after each procedure, using the same criteria as in a surgical center.

- Special situation: there is a type of applicator, the cylinder, which doesn't require fasting or anesthesia, because its insertion is not painful. Insertion of the bladder catheter and the X-ray also only take place when it is first inserted.

Nurse competencies in brachytherapy:

- Participating in the process of scheduling clients for the procedure, checking if there are any obstacles to it taking place and working with the interdisciplinary team to solve problems.

- The management of the treatment room is essential for carrying out the procedures. The nurse must supply the room with materials and check that the equipment is working properly, notifying the secretary of any defects. The nurse is also responsible for preparing the room and setting up the trays to be used.

- The care of the applicators is the responsibility of the nurses in the sector. According to the hospital's routine, after the procedures they are washed, packaged and delivered to the sector secretaries, who arrange for them to be sent to INCA for ethylene oxide sterilization. In the event of any problems, the nurses will have to contact the doctors and department secretaries to find the appropriate solutions together. All this is done to ensure that the material is fit for use.

- Five types of applicators are used in gynecological brachytherapy: Martinez, colpostate with tanden, ring, cylinder with tanden and isolated cylinder. It is the nurse's responsibility to assemble the applicators when preparing the tray.

- Nursing consultations for clients undergoing brachytherapy should take place before the first application, for guidance on the treatment, and after the last application, for guidance on post-treatment care.

- Comprehensive care for the client undergoing gynecological brachytherapy is the responsibility of the department nurse, as is action in the event of complications. Don't forget that the nursing team is an important reference point for the client, especially while she (the client) is in the room.

- For clients who have undergone prolonged fasting, food is provided through the Nutrition Service.

- Nursing technicians must assist the nurse in the comprehensive care of the clients, as well as in the care of the equipment and the room. They can also assist the radiotherapist and anesthesiologist, if necessary.

- The anesthesia used in this type of procedure is sedation. It is the nurse's responsibility to have the anesthesia trolley checked for functionality and the supply of controlled medication. At HUCFF, there are anesthesia technicians who perform this function. This is an essential task, since any anesthesia procedure carried out outside the operating room becomes more complex, and the healthcare team must plan safely for this activity (DENARDI et al, 2008).

Routine brachytherapy procedure at the hospital in Barretos

The Barretos Cancer Hospital also uses the Iridium[192] source to treat gynecological brachytherapy. The aspects that differ from the routine at the hospital in Rio de Janeiro will be described. For the rest, the procedures are carried out in a similar way in both institutions. The following information was kindly provided by the team of nurses at the Barretos hospital and is included in their manual of rules and routines, which was drawn up by Vanzelli, Carvalho and Lima (2009).

The Barretos institution's protocol for clients with a clinical diagnosis of uterine and vaginal cancer includes external radiotherapy (teletherapy) and internal radiotherapy (brachytherapy), carried out concurrently. Clients undergo two brachytherapy sessions a week, so that the treatment lasts fifteen days. If necessary, chemotherapy is also administered during this period. This is because most of the clients come from distant regions, such as Rondonia, Acre, Mato Grosso, Mato Grosso do Sul, Minas Gerais and Goias. Therefore, by shortening treatment, it becomes possible for these clients to return to their place of origin more quickly, as well as creating possibilities for treating a greater number of clients in a shorter space of time.

It should be emphasized that, in this way, the treatment takes on a rigorous aspect, and care for these clients is intensified, with proper monitoring by the multidisciplinary team.

According to the aforementioned authors (Vanzelli and Lima, 2009), these are the aspects that differentiate the routine in the two scenarios in this study:

- At the Barretos hospital, the nursing technicians take care of the clients directly in the room. The room is managed by the nurses.

- Anesthesia is performed on medical advice. Therefore, not all clients are anesthetized. Those who are not, receive common intravenous analgesia before the procedure.

- General cleaning of the room is only carried out at the beginning and end of the working day. In between procedures, the hygiene and cleaning team acts if necessary.

- Clients are scheduled by the nursing technicians in partnership with the doctors. Guidance on the treatment is given by the nurse during the consultation prior to the teletherapy and before the brachytherapy begins. On the day of the procedure, the nursing technician in the room can reinforce the instructions.

- Only clients who need anesthesia need to be fasting.

- Ultrasound is used to visualize when the applicator is inserted, and a device is available in the room for this purpose.

- Nursing technicians can remove the applicator and the bladder catheter, as they have been trained in this activity beforehand.

- The nursing technician is the one who releases the client. In the event of any complications, the presence of the nurse is requested in the room.

- The nursing technicians order the material for use in the room. The nurse checks the material in and out. The room and trays are prepared by the nursing technicians.

- Caring for the applicators is the responsibility of nurses and nursing technicians.

- After use, the material is placed in a sodium sulphite solution (cidex cepa) for sterilization, as instructed by the hospital's Infection Control Committee. It is rinsed with saline solution. The material is left in the solution for forty minutes.

- When anesthesia is administered, the anesthesiologist assesses the client and spinal anesthesia is the option used.

In view of the above, nursing's participation in this type of procedure is notorious. The institutions mentioned in this study follow the principles of the literature on the role of nursing in brachytherapy. Thus, according to Denardi et al (2008), nurses must work with the multidisciplinary team, ensuring that the treatment is carried out, that clients receive the necessary guidance and that side effects are managed. Also according to the authors, it is important for nurses to assist clients directly during the procedure in question, guarantee their privacy and help the multidisciplinary team to control radiological protection measures.

4. THE NURSING CONSULTATION IN BRACHYTHERAPY

This chapter describes how the nursing consultation is carried out for clients undergoing brachytherapy at the hospital in Rio de Janeiro. The nursing consultation for brachytherapy at the hospital in Barretos takes place in a similar way.

THE NURSING CONSULTATION IN BRACHYTHERAPY

I agree with Micozzi (2008) that the structure of nursing care can come from the body of knowledge of other disciplines, such as sociology, anthropology, philosophy, psychology, among others. This gives nurses a professional identity and contributes to the profession's body of knowledge. And this range of knowledge qualifies nurses for the nursing consultation (NC), as it prepares them to care for the client holistically. Therefore, according to Vanzin and Nery (2000), nursing, due to its training, is the **only** team within any health system that is uniquely qualified to care for clients twenty-four hours a day.

This activity (CE) provides the opportunity to teach and learn, in an exchange of experiences between those who care and those who are cared for. The empathy that arises between clients and nurses is subjective, but it can help to identify evidence that will help to plan appropriate care for that individual.

This integration of evidence with the clinical experience of the nurse and the characteristics of the clients is important because it forms the basis of the advice given in consultations, which must have individual meaning for the client (BORK, 2005).

Vanzin and Nery (2000) tell us that

Nursing consultation is the systematic and continuous care provided to individuals, families and communities by professional nurses with the aim of promoting health through early diagnosis and treatment.

According to Rosas (1998), the nursing consultation should be personalized, based on the needs of each individual, noting their uniqueness and the meaning it has for them.

It is a private activity of the nurse, according to the Law of Professional Nursing Practice No. 7.498 of 25/06/86, regulated by Decree No. 94406 of 08/06/87, and cannot be delegated. It uses scientific methods to identify disease situations and prescribe nursing measures that contribute to the promotion of health, with a view to preventing illness and recovering the individual's health (BRASIL, COFEN, 2009). It is therefore an educational activity.

In the case of clients undergoing brachytherapy at the HUCFF Radiotherapy Department, we try to establish a relationship of trust, empathy and familiarity, so that they can really interact with the nurse. We mustn't forget that we are dealing with these clients' private issues, and it won't always be easy for them to expose their privacy. This empathy in the nursing consultation is very well described by Rosas (2003), when he emphasizes the importance of the professional's interaction with the clients during the consultation.

As already mentioned, at HUCFF, the nursing consultation for brachytherapy treatment takes place before the first application and after the last. When it is decided by the radiotherapist that the client should undergo the treatment in question, she is referred to the nursing department immediately after the consultation with the doctor. From then on, clients are instructed on the steps of the procedure and care before, during and after brachytherapy applications.

The precautions that must be taken before each application are:

- If anesthesia is necessary, fast for eight hours.

- In the case of clients taking medication for chronic illnesses, the only medication that can be taken on an empty stomach is antihypertensive medication, with as little water as possible, in order to prevent the fear of treatment from raising blood pressure. In the case of clients taking oral hypoglycemic agents or insulin, advise them **not to** take the medication, as they will be fasting for a long time and could develop hypoglycemia if they are under the effect. We usually pay extra attention to clients who use both types of medication, emphasizing which one to take and which one not to take. The other medications can be taken immediately after treatment.

- Trim the pubic hair or trichotomy the genital area.

- Attend accompanied, as it is recommended that outpatients undergoing anesthesia should not be released from the hospital alone after the procedure (BRASIL, MS, 2001; ASA, 2009).

- Do not use cream or any medication vaginally two days before application, in order to spare the area that will receive the treatment.

- Explain the possible need to remove the prosthesis. As this could lead to embarrassment for the client, explain that the prosthesis will be removed in the treatment room, just before the procedure, and that the client should spend as little time as possible without her prosthesis.

- Do not attend treatment wearing dark nail polish, so that it does not interfere with the health team's view of the color of the nail bed.

- No cream on the skin around the genital area.

The recommended precautions during treatment are:

- Avoid the use of vaginal creams in the periods close to application.

- Advise them to drink plenty of fluids in order to avoid urinary infection, as constant hydration of the urinary tract dilutes the urine, thus reducing the chances of this type of infection. An abundant liquid intake also hydrates the intestine, helping it to function properly. Pay attention to the cases of clients with dietary restrictions.

- Ask the client how she is feeling as the treatment progresses. Ask about pain, vaginal bleeding and vaginal discharge. An assessment of the client's general condition is recommended before each application.

The recommended care after the four applications is as follows:

Advising the client on:

- Returning to your original doctor.

- Routine gynecological preventive examinations should be carried out six months after the end of treatment, in accordance with the institutional protocol.

- The vaginal dilation exercise is used to prevent stenosis, a common side effect of the treatment. In this case, the client should perform the exercise with a prepared syringe, provided by the ward nurse, or have sexual relations with a partner.

Any of these activities should be carried out with a condom to protect the area that has been treated. Preventing vaginal stenosis and stiffening is important because, if this occurs, it will be difficult to perform the gynecological preventive exam. This is because the exam involves a bimanual examination of the pelvis and the placement of a vaginal speculum (SILVA, GANNUNY, AIELLO, HIGINIO, FERREIRA, OLIVEIRA, 2010; BRASIL, MS INCA, 2012).

It is essential to emphasize that some women, even today, find it difficult to talk about their private lives. Therefore, talking about the uterus, vagina and sexual relations tends to be an embarrassing task, especially for older clients. The empathy needed for this can be achieved with affection and respect (FIGUEIREDO et al, 2009).

Gynecological brachytherapy for clients with psychiatric disorders can only be carried out with the written consent of their family member or guardian, as they are considered to be a vulnerable group. Clients who have never had sexual intercourse must also authorize the procedure in writing, so that it does not constitute bodily harm.

5. TEACHING AND LEARNING IN THE NURSING CONSULTATION (NC) ACTIVITY

This chapter deals with the teaching-learning process that takes place in the nursing consultation.

TEACHING AND LEARNING IN NURSING CONSULTATIONS

It is gratifying to realize that today's clients are becoming demanding consumers of the health system. The promotion and maintenance of health has become a subject of interest to the population, going beyond the goals of disease prevention. With the increase in chronic health conditions, people increasingly want to learn how to take better care of themselves, modifying behaviors considered to be risky in order to reduce complications (BASTABLE, 2010).

The nursing consultation establishes a process of interaction, stimulating self-care. This activity must be efficient for both the person being cared for and the caregiver. Listening to the client, accepting them and forming a therapeutic alliance are important tasks when carrying out a NC. As a result, good self-care practices emerge, which are attitudes aimed at the client's comfort and well-being (LOPES, SILVEIRA, e FERREIRA, 1999). Therefore, in order for the client to accept the guidance provided by the nurse, it is necessary for the professional to take into account the client's experience and impressions of life and what this guidance means to them (the client).

Trezza (2002), in her thesis, defines the human being as a unique person, each with their own way of getting sick and healing. Thus, still referring to the author, it is up to the nurse to help the client find their (the client's) way of living with the illness and coping with it. Therefore, the nurse's role in the client's healing process is fundamental. And the educational activities developed with the client are part of this.

This is the teaching and learning movement. Education enlightens and helps the person, making it a powerful tool, including helping the learner to protect themselves from possible abuse (BASTABLE, 2010). It is believed that every client has the right to appropriate information, especially when it comes to cancer clients. This is so that they don't feel misled during their therapeutic process. I emphasize that every treatment process in oncology is long and brings physical and emotional suffering for as long as it lasts.

Nurses' role as educators is extremely important. After all, educating is one of the ways of caring for others. Whenever we teach, we are caring. And whenever we are caring, we can use this moment with the client and their family to teach. Due to their training, nurses have great potential for guiding clients and should make the most of this ability (VANZIN & NERY, 2000; GATES & FINK et al, 2009; BASTABLE, 2010).

Nurses and clients are alike, attracted by common interests: caring and being cared for. That said, if the professional is able to grasp the client's experience in its entirety, empathy is established, which will help in drawing up an effective care plan.

This type of exchange can be called intersubjectivity, which happens when the interested parties understand each other (SCHUTZ, 2012). There is no need for ascendancy or authoritarianism. It's a partnership, driven by the same reason. When educating through nursing consultations, it should be borne in mind that this process is individual to each human being. In short, students learn what they want, the way they want, at their own pace. Nothing should be imposed in order for the educational process to truly take place.

In the nursing consultation activity, nurses can both plan the client's discharge from hospital and plan outpatient care, optimizing the client's independence. Everything that is taught and learned in the ND can have repercussions on the client's treatment as a whole, changing the client's experience of self-care and the nurse's experience of care. For this reason, the nursing consultation is recognized as an educational process.

As nurses are the health providers closest to their clients, they must be approachable and trustworthy. This justifies the need for empathy between the professional providing care and the person receiving it. It is understood that in the teaching-learning relationship there must be a commitment on both sides: there must be someone who wants to teach and someone who wants to learn. And when you think about the needs of the individual as a whole, you have to make sure that it was possible to meet their educational demands (ROSAS, 2003; GATES & FINK et al, 2009; SANTOS, 2009; BASTABLE, 2010).

Below are some of the criteria identified as fundamental for the realization of CE, according to Rosas (2003), Santos (2009), Bastable (2010) and Saraiva (2011):

- Approach the person holistically. Cultural issues are equally important and must not be forgotten.

- Take into account the special conditions of the clients. EC should be designed to take into account the uniqueness of everyone, even in situations where the approach is more difficult, such as in cases of physical and/or mental limitations. It is important that everyone has access to the benefits of EC.

- Partner with the client's family or social network. They can be strong allies for the healthcare team in the care process.

- Providing explanatory leaflets that are easy for clients to understand. This strengthens the teaching-learning process that takes place at the EC.

- Try to maintain an empathetic relationship with your clients. This helps in the moment of exchange, when you teach your clients and learn from them, and also encourages them to become aware of how important efficient self-care is.

- Prescribe care within the client's reality. Only in this way will the planned activities become achievable. Distinguish common sense from absurdity. It is not uncommon for non-adherence to guidelines to be interpreted as rebellion, when in fact it is impossible to follow them. With regard to this, Santos (2003) says that the learning content must be meaningful to the learner and related to their personal experiences. The client must have the power to decide, and the last word must belong to them.

- Don't judge the clientele. Educating is an exchange, and for this it is necessary to respect the other person's uniqueness and worldview, without value judgments.

- Care with privacy and secrecy. The lived experience of others must also be respected.

- Learning to learn from clients. It must be admitted that nurses have a lot to learn from their clients. You must be attentive to every possibility of exchange.

- Remember that in CE there must be a mutual interest, which is education. To educate is to relate to the other, to match motives and intentions. It is desirable that the nurse's teaching plan meets the client's learning needs.

- Guiding the client's movement within the health unit, helping in cases of doubt whenever possible.

- Repeat the information as many times as necessary. The client may be nervous about absorbing what is said at the time.

- Establish priorities. Teach what is necessary for the moment.

- Provide guidance on several occasions. The client may not be able to absorb a great deal of information in a single interview.

With this beiKic teaching and learning for clients and nurses, we can share experiences, knowledge and dialogues, which makes us greater as people. I agree with Bastable (2010) when he says that this type of exchange of experience, which is the educational process, is a permanent cycle in the life of the human being, present in both the personal and professional fields. So is phenomenology, since living is a unique experience with its own meaning for each person (SCHUTZ, 2012).

It is known that the main objective of EC is to promote and maintain health, with the aim of enabling clients to exploit their self-care potential to the full (VANZIN and NERY, 2000). In the case of clients undergoing gynecological brachytherapy, the aim is to make them experience the treatment in the best possible way. The teaching and learning that EC provides is such a rich exchange that it is difficult to say who is teaching and who is learning.

In this sector (HUCFF/UFRJ), consultations are personalized, since each client is unique. We tried to define the reasons for the care based on the reasons the clients had for coming to the EC, in order to guarantee their independence. The important thing is to make sure that they follow the advice given and cope with treatment in a satisfactory way. The partnership that emerges between everyone involved in the nursing consultation can also make it easier for family members to understand and follow the therapy. In this phase, which is so difficult for clients, friends and family help to structure care by collaborating with them. This is why they are included in the treatment process.

When necessary, specific strategies are adopted for special situations in order to overcome limitations. After all, we want the care process to be resolutive. Nursing consultations for clients undergoing gynecological brachytherapy at HUCFF are tailored to their reality. Guidance is tailored to their life routine and is provided in a democratic way, so that it has a positive impact.

The sharing of knowledge and experiences that takes place during EC helps to modify behavior. This increases the chances of improving the quality of life of clients undergoing treatment, as well as increasing the chances of improving the standard of care offered.

As nurses have prolonged contact with clients in healthcare facilities, they should be present whenever possible. Through guidance, they have the opportunity to facilitate positive changes in their clients' lives, using the potential of the profession to share knowledge. When nurses interact, they join clients and their families, sometimes as facilitators and sometimes as learners. And this teaching and learning helps to understand the clients' universe, leading to a planning of care that is close to the ideal.

Teaching and learning with clients in the gynecological brachytherapy procedure:

Gynecological brachytherapy began at the hospital where I work (HUCFF) in 2007. Initially, there was no nursing consultation for these clients, as the service was in the process of building a protocol for this activity and because the flow of clients in the sector was still being defined. The ideal time for them to be taken to the EC had yet to be decided. Finally, it was agreed with the department secretaries (who book the appointments) and the radiotherapy doctors that the consultation with the nurse should take place immediately after the doctor's appointment, when the client was told that she needed to undergo gynecological brachytherapy.

From then on, this routine was established, and EC was considered an automatic event in the sector immediately after the medical consultation. This made it possible for these clients and their families to be instructed on what would happen during the procedure, how they should act and what care they should take of themselves before, during and after the treatment (which lasts approximately one month).

After the routine was implemented, we saw the benefits of EC for these clients. They arrived at the ward less apprehensive and more collaborative. They were fully capable of self-care and showed that they understood the advice they received. Effective self-care helps to reduce the undesirable effects of treatment. This also allows for a more peaceful anesthesia induction and an excellent post-procedure recovery.

Teaching and learning between clients and nurses, when it comes to gynecological brachytherapy, begins during the nursing consultation. The interaction begins with clarifying everything that will happen to the client during the procedure. After all, this is an invasive procedure and, even if the client has been informed about it beforehand, she may still be doubtful and anxious.

Rosa and Sales (2008) point out that the medical literature doesn't describe exactly what it means for the client to undergo this type of treatment and that the healthcare team lacks the necessary attention to provide detailed guidance about the procedure. Thus, it is understood that the technical information described in the literature is important, but concern for the client's emotional state is also fundamental.

I emphasize that we are talking about cancer. Even with the technology available today, statistics show that the disease still has an uncertain prognosis, based solely on disease-free time (BRASIL, MS, INCA, 2012). The stigma of death hangs over the approaches, even if it is implicit, since it is a chronic degenerative disease that affects people in different ways, and it is difficult to base oneself on just one pattern of reflection when it comes to it.

In view of the above, it is essential to establish a relationship with the client in which she can express herself freely, trying to resolve her doubts and making her willing to self-care, without losing hope for the future. Below, we describe some of the elements present in the nursing consultation for clients undergoing gynecological brachytherapy, as a result of the practice of care. These factors can be of concern to clients.

Their perspective on anesthesia, knowing that they will be sedated and lose consciousness, is not usually the most pleasant. Nurses teach when they explain what the procedure will be like and how clients should prepare for it. And they learn when they tell them how they feel during the gynecological brachytherapy sessions and how they take care of themselves during the treatment period. Also in agreement with Rosa and Sales (2008), I believe that it is the nurse's responsibility to identify this moment of fragility in the clients and ensure that they go through the treatment without trauma.

At the start of the nursing consultation, you should be aware of the client's ability to have a conversation about the treatment. If she is preoccupied with a bureaucratic problem, pain, family problems or excessive fear of the procedure, these factors could prevent her from understanding gynecological brachytherapy and how she should take care of herself. Nurses need to be sensitive to recognizing how to establish this exchange, assessing the subjectivity of the situation. After all, the relationship between client and professional must be beneficial and productive for both; a positive face-to-face relationship.

Some issues of a personal nature are addressed in the consultation prior to gynecological brachytherapy. The client's sexual activity and the vaginal dilation exercise can be embarrassing subjects. Borges (2003), in her master's dissertation, explains how upsetting it can be to broach the subject with the client, since, knowing she is ill, she (the client) may not want to reflect on her sexuality.

Therefore, before mentioning the subject, the nurse needs to signal to the client that there is a moment in the nursing consultation when she might prefer to be alone with the professional. There are clients who report being abandoned by their spouse because of their illness. This could be another reason why they don't want to talk about sexuality. Teaching clients means supporting them and guiding them through these aspects. Learning with them means identifying what to talk about in the presence of family/friends. It's important to respect their individuality.

In the course of the practice, it was found that the clients value technical information about self-care. As for the nurses, what each client says helps the professional to understand the universe of the others, because although they are all unique, there are situations that are repeated. Knowing the cultural background of the clients is gratifying, as it helps to establish a relationship of understanding. I agree with Barbosa, Teixeira and Pereira (2007) when they emphasize the importance of combining the technical knowledge of nurses with the popular knowledge of clients in order to provide efficient care.

According to Panobianco, Pimentel, Almeida and Oliveira (2012), the nursing consultation is an opportunity to teach and learn from the clients. Health education can create an opportunity to improve these clients' understanding of the disease, generating coping strategies with positive results and increased adherence to treatment.

This sharing of knowledge is useful, leading to the understanding that when clients don't adhere to treatment, it's not always because they don't want to, but because they don't have the socio-cultural structure to follow these guidelines. Thus, in the sectors mentioned in this study, the idea of what is in common between the clients will give the intentionality of the nurse's actions for care. One of the products of this study is the establishment of a flexible protocol, so that the experience and uniqueness of each client is respected. Flexibility will be present when we understand that bringing together the different singularities of the clients will lead to their typical, to the common points between them. From these points, the bases for the reconstruction of the aforementioned protocol are being extracted.

Bastable (2010) states that learning takes place when information becomes knowledge. From there, the individual is transformed and adheres to what has been taught. This is what aims to achieve when sharing knowledge with clients during nursing consultations. In this way, nurses continue to teach by learning. And the clients learn by teaching.

6. THEORETICAL-METHODOLOGICAL FRAMEWORK

This chapter discusses the theoretical-methodological framework on which the study is based: the

Alfred Schutz's Sociological Phenomenology.

THEORETICAL-METHODOLOGICAL FRAMEWORK

The phenomenological approach was used to ground and guide the study. Phenomenology is a philosophical movement that studies the essence of the phenomenon, describing every experience as it is (MARTINS & BICUDO, 1983). It focuses on the meaning that people give to the facts of life. It is a line of thought based on people's life experiences and what their experiences represent to them, understanding how the phenomenon is lived (SCHUTZ, 1979, 2012).

In this sense, considering that each of us has our own way of seeing the world, it is understood that phenomenology wants to know how the individual is incorporated into it. It is a philosophical movement that aims to understand people through the way things happen to them in the world of life (SCHUTZ, 1979, 2012).

This is a descriptive study with a qualitative, exploratory approach, working with the universe of meaning and motivations, something that cannot be quantified. The choice of reference, Alfred Schutz's Sociological Phenomenology, was due to the recognition of the importance of the baggage of knowledge that each client and nurse carries within themselves, understanding that every nursing consultation is an opportunity for learning, the result of the interpersonal relationships of this encounter.

Phenomenology was created by Edmund Husserl (1859-1938) in Germany in the 19th century as a reaction to positivist empiricism. It arose from the need for scientists to explain phenomena logically, without the rigorous pragmatism of positivism. Husserl had several followers, such as Heidegger (1889-1976), who studied phenomenology through the meaning of being; Merleau Ponty (1908-1961), who focused on the body and consciousness as perception and Schutz, who dedicated himself to the intentionality of the action of being, manifested through its motives (CAPALBO, 1998, 2008).

Alfred Schutz, a lawyer and sociologist who was born in Vienna in 1899 and died in New York in 1959, proposed concepts in his sociological phenomenology that help us understand social action. Some of these are: the lived, meaning, subjectivity, intersubjectivity, singularity and intentionality (SCHUTZ, 1979, 2012).

For the author, every experience (**lived**) has a **meaning** for each individual and the perception of this experience is unique, since each human being is unique. **Subjectivity** refers to everything that belongs to the subject (person). **Intersubjectivity** appears when we leave our world and look at the other, in an exchange of experience - it's **me and you** (SCHUTZ, 1979, 2012).

With regard to **intentionality**, there are conceptions that reveal that human beings act according to motivations aimed at objectives. These are motives-for and motives-why. According to Schutz (1962, p.71),

The motive-for refers to the attitude of the actor experiencing the process of their developing action. It is therefore an essentially subjective category and is only revealed to the observer when they ask what meaning the actor gives to their action.

Thus, the motives for action are related to the future. The subject of the action can imagine it, he mentally anticipates his conduct, according to his intentions (SCHUTZ, 1979, 2012).

[1] Reasons-why refer to the past, and Schutz (1962, p. 72) tells us that:

The motive-why is an objective category, accessible to the observer who must reconstruct the actor's attitude towards his act from the completed act. It is only when the actor turns to his past, and thus becomes an observer of his own actions, that he can grasp the genuine motive behind his actions.

In light of the above, the motives-why explain the act that was completed; they explain the path taken from the motives-for to the motives-why (Schutz, 2012). Understanding that the **motives-for** explain the reasons that determine the individual's behavior and the **motives-why** refer to the context of the event that occurred, the aim of this study is to adapt the intentionality of the care provided by nurses to the reasons that clients have for coming to the health unit for treatment. In order to do this, it will be necessary to know how clients position themselves in the face of treatment and how nurses position themselves in the face of care, as will be explained below.

With regard to the clients, I was interested in learning about their experiences of the disease and its impact on their **lives**. I tried to find out what the illness **meant** to them, the proposed treatment and the fact that they had nursing consultations at their disposal. Thus, **subjectivity and intersubjectivity** emerged in the act of sharing experiences, in the exchanges that took place during the nursing consultations. **Uniqueness** became evident when I realized that treatment affects each client in a certain way. And this particular worldview can be the starting point for structuring care.

With regard to the nurses, I was interested in getting to know their experience (their **lived experience)** with the practice of nursing consultation; how they perceive the situation of clients undergoing brachytherapy. I wanted to know what **it means** for them to share teaching and learning with their clients, in an **intersubjective** relationship, during nursing consultations. The **uniqueness** was evident when we realized that each consultation is a unique moment, including the way in which the person is guided. Therefore, just as the nursing consultation is unique for each client, it is also unique for nurses, and the way they look at each client is different.

Capalbo (2008), when he tells us about the need to understand the experience of the other, reinforces the importance of behavior being understood, because this understanding makes social coexistence possible. When it comes to nursing consultations, understanding the other person helps in the practice of care, since by getting to know clients as a whole, you can define what their needs are.

In this sense, Schutz (1979, 2012) states that the experience of human beings explains their **motivations**, their **intentionality**. In this study, the aim was to interweave the nurses' motivations with those of the clients. The basis of the reconstruction of the protocol that I have in mind will come from the clients' reasons for experiencing the proposed treatment, added to the nurses' reasons for promoting care. And this will be possible by getting to know the teaching and learning process that takes place between the two during the nursing consultation.

In view of the above, Alfred Schutz's Sociological Phenomenology was suitable as a basis for this study, since the framework deals with questions of the uniqueness of the human being, backed up by their baggage of knowledge, which constitutes elements that help in understanding the needs of others.

METHODOLOGICAL PATHS.

The study scenarios:

The thesis was carried out in two settings: the Radiotherapy Department of the Clementino Fraga Filho University Hospital, a general, public, university hospital located in Rio de Janeiro, and the Radiotherapy Department of the Barretos Cancer Hospital, a philanthropic hospital specializing in oncology, located in the same city. Both institutions primarily serve clients of the Unified Health System, receiving people from all over Brazil for treatment.

The HUCFF is maintained by the Federal Government and serves a significant number of clients from the state of Rio de Janeiro, the northeast and southeast of the country. The Hospital de Cancer de Barretos, of the Pio XII Foundation, has donations as its main source of income and serves a significant number of clients from the state of São Paulo, the center of the country and the south-east.

west and north of the country. The PIO XII Foundation also maintains several support houses to accommodate clients from other states, since cancer treatment takes place over a long period of time. Clients are guaranteed airfare and accommodation.

In both hospitals, clients undergoing brachytherapy treatment are referred from teletherapy, following the following flow: **oncology - radiotherapy - brachytherapy - oncology**.

The HUCFF Radiotherapy Department has a linear accelerator (for teletherapy) and an Iridium[192] source. This sector is located on two floors. The first floor houses the treatment equipment and the second floor houses the consultations. On each floor there is a rest room with a stretcher for clients who need some care.

The nursing team is made up of three nurses and four nursing technicians, with one nurse and two nursing technicians working per shift. The third nurse works every day in the morning, taking on the tasks of management and nursing care in the sector. Teaching and research activities are the responsibility of the three nurses. Any member of the nursing team is assigned to work in both teletherapy and brachytherapy.

At the Barretos Cancer Hospital, brachytherapy treatment is scheduled to last around fifteen days. The Radiotherapy Department at this hospital also has two floors. The upper floor houses the administrative area. On the lower floor, there are ten consulting rooms, a rest room with a capacity for six beds, six teletherapy machines and an iridium source[192]. The nursing team consists of three nurses (two nurses and one nurse) and twelve nursing technicians. The nurses are per diem, with the responsibility of managing the care, acting in it and developing teaching and research activities.

The subjects of the study:

The study included female clients over the age of eighteen who were lucid and oriented, undergoing gynecological brachytherapy and the nurses from the sectors in question. As **inclusion criteria**, clients who so wished participated in the study, regardless of the stage of the clinical diagnosis or the length of treatment. The general condition of the interviewees was not a concern, since only healthy clients undergo brachytherapy. With regard to the nurses, those who work with clients undergoing gynecological brachytherapy and provide nursing consultations for these clients took part in the study, regardless of how long they have been in the profession or how long they have been working in this field.

The **exclusion criteria** were initially left to the people interviewed (this rule applied to both clients and nurses): they depended on their desire to take part in the study. Clients with pain, bleeding or any other physical or emotional discomfort were not invited to take part. The meetings were held by appointment, for the convenience of the interviewees. The interviews with the nurses took place according to their time availability, and all of them kindly agreed to take part in the study.

Ethical aspects of the study:

Authorizations were requested and granted from the clients, the nurses and the Research Ethics Committees (CEPs) of the hospitals in question, in compliance with Resolution 196/96 of the National Health Council, which deals with the rules for research with human beings. The study was approved and registered at the HUCFF under number 127/11 and at the Barretos Cancer Hospital under number 551/2011. Authorizations were also requested from the immediate heads of the sectors in question, and the Nurse Coordinator of the Barretos Cancer Hospital became the researcher's representative before this institution.

The anonymity of the study subjects was guaranteed by replacing the interviewees' names with color names. This decision was made because each color is unique, with an equally unique meaning for each individual. Therefore, the subjectivity of each color will represent in the study the subjectivity of each individual's testimony. All the people interviewed agreed to change their names, leaving it up to the researcher to choose the colors.

Field stages:

With regard to the nurses at HUCFF, where I work, I asked them to participate during working hours, as I share the same schedule. The interviews took place on scheduled dates, according to the nurses' demand for services. With regard to the nurses at the Barretos Cancer Hospital, their participation in the study was confirmed during the technical visit and ambience. I considered it necessary to visit the hospital so that I could get to know the hospital's routine and collect data without interfering in the work structure, since I am not an employee of the institution. The interviews also took place by appointment, according to the nurses' demand for services.

With regard to the clients, I used a similar approach for both institutions: requesting their cooperation when they were in their third or fourth application of the treatment, and scheduling the date of the interview according to their convenience. I chose to interview the clients after the third or fourth application, as this is a phase near the end of the treatment, when the clients are already familiar with it and one more activity (in this case, the interview) would not be a nuisance for them.

All the interviews took place on a scheduled day, time and place. The locations of the interviews were the consulting rooms where the nursing consultations take place. The nursing consulting rooms at both institutions were set up to conduct the interviews in comfort and privacy. The same method was used in both institutions.

Speeches were recorded and then transcribed. The data obtained was used only for this study. The recording equipment is in my possession to guarantee the confidentiality of the information. The recordings will be erased from the device's media five years after the end of the study, in accordance with CNS law 196/96. An MP4 device was used for this purpose. No images of the research subjects were used.

The data was analyzed based on the most frequently encountered concerns, i.e. the analysis of categories established from there. As this is a phenomenological study, I used the expressive meanings of each of the interviewees as a basis. This number was defined by the feeling of closure, when new data began to produce repeated information. I therefore interviewed thirteen clients.

The number of nurses interviewed was defined differently: I wanted to hear all the professionals from the two institutions, two in RJ and four in Barretos. One nurse in SP was a Nursing Resident at the time of the study. In all, six interviews were conducted.

In order to analyze the statements, I worked with subjective data, i.e. the subjects' reflections on the expectations of teaching and learning in the nursing consultation for clients undergoing gynecological brachytherapy. Data collection followed these steps:

- Technical visit to the Barretos Cancer Hospital. This practice was important as both the author and the study supervisor live in Rio de Janeiro. There was no need to visit the institution in Rio de Janeiro, as it is where I work.

- Scheduling the interviews (date, place and time - in both scenarios).

- Recorded interviews (in both scenarios).

- The interviews were transcribed, keeping the original speech so as not to lose their subjectivity.

- Reading and analysis of transcripts.

- **Apprehension of the meaning of** the speeches.

- Organization of clients' and nurses' speeches according to their motivations.

- Definition of speech categories.

- Comprehensive analysis of the speeches, in the light of Alfred Schutz's Sociological Phenomenology.

Three visits were made to the Barretos Cancer Hospital: the first for the environment and the following two for the interviews. Prior contact had been made with the nurse coordinator of the department, by telephone and email, and she was informed about the study and agreed to it.

The first visit to the institution consisted of several moments: first, I personally presented the study to the nurse coordinator of the Radiotherapy Department, obtaining written authorization from those responsible for the sector to carry it out. Afterwards, I contacted the hospital's Ethics Committee team in person, finalizing the delivery of the documentation that had been started over the internet. Next, I made a technical visit to the Radiotherapy Department, where I met the multidisciplinary team that works there. Finally, I accompanied the gynecological brachytherapy procedures and nursing consultations for clients undergoing this type of treatment.

It is important to note that the environment helped to define the strategy for attracting clients for the interview, as well as helping to familiarize them with the routine and the health team in the sector. Since this is a study based on Phenomenology, this experience was necessary in order to establish an empathetic relationship with both the clients and the professional team, leading to a face-to-face relationship. The aim was to carry out the interviews with the minimum of interference in the sector's routine. This practice both complied with the method of the study and made it more comfortable for the subjects to take part in it.

To obtain the data, an open-ended, unstructured interview was used, which, according to Polit, Beck & Hungler (2004), consists of allowing the interviewee to speak freely about the proposed topic, without being interrupted. Thus, clients and nurses were able to freely narrate their experience of the nursing consultation and how they perceive brachytherapy treatment.

We used the concepts of the phenomenological interview by Carvalho (1991). According to the author, this type of interview captures the person's way of experiencing the world, taking into account their values and experiences. This can be achieved when there is communion between the speaker and the listener. Also according to Carvalho (1991), in order to achieve the objective of the phenomenological interview, the interviewer must set aside their own ideas in order to consider the ideas of the interviewee. The interviewer must distance themselves from their own experience, abandoning their own value judgments in order to reach the meaning of the other person's experience. It's about empathy, putting yourself in the other person's shoes.

Considering the empathy required for a phenomenological interview, it can be said that it has the necessary requirements for its realization. Carvalho (1991) states that in order to capture the client's way of experiencing the world, the interview must take place in a private environment, without external interference. The gestures, gaze and tone of voice of the person speaking must be taken into account in order to understand the other person's thoughts. The interviewer should maintain a receptive posture, but without showing signs of their own opinion, so as not to influence the response of the interviewee.

That said, the above-mentioned technique guided the interviews. The questions used were:

For customers:

- What do you have in mind when it comes to EC brachytherapy?

- How do you experience teaching and learning in brachytherapy treatment?

- Tell us what it has meant to you to teach and learn with EC in brachytherapy treatment.

For nurses:

- Tell us how you plan and carry out the nursing consultation in brachytherapy treatment.

- What do you have in mind when you teach and learn from your clients in the nursing consultation during brachytherapy treatment?

- What does it mean for you to teach and learn from clients during CE in brachytherapy treatment?

The interviewees were also asked about some of their biographical data, such as:

- In the case of the clients: length of cancer treatment, age, education, profession and whether they have ever suffered from a gynecological disease.

- In the case of nurses: degree, time since graduation and how long they have been working in brachytherapy, performing the CE activity.

The answers obtained from the clients and the nurses provided input for the development of some categories that reflect the intentionality of the interviewees' actions regarding the nursing consultation in gynecological brachytherapy. The aim was to get to know the lived experiences of the clients who undergo brachytherapy and the nurses who work in these sectors, so that the care is appropriate to the needs signaled by the subjects of the study.

7. DEVELOPING COMPREHENSIVE ANALYSIS IN THE LIGHT OF ALFRED SCHUTZ'S SOCIOLOGICAL PHENOMENOLOGY

This chapter describes how the comprehensive analysis was developed. According to the proposed framework, categories emerged from the subjects' common statements and described their type of experience.

COMPREHENSIVE ANALYSIS

I obtained expressive meanings from the subjects' statements, which contributed to the formation of categories. In all, thirteen clients and six nurses were interviewed. The following tables provide data on the biographical situation of the subjects of this thesis:

Biographical data of clients:

Codename	Age	Instruction	Born in	Occupation	Profession	Treatment time
White	30	Middle school	PA	Home		05 months
Lilas	69	Complete primary education	RJ	Home		08 months
Grena	34	Elementary school incomplete	RJ	Home		09 months
Red	52	Middle school	SP		Merchant	01 year
Yellow	63	High school incomplete	MG	Home		01 year
Blue	76	Complete primary education	SP		Retired housewife	11 months

Coral	38	Complete primary education	RO		Farmer	03 months
Graphite	67	Middle school	SP		Retired seamstress	10 months
Cream	46	Complete primary education	AC		Domestic	09 months
Caramel	59	Middle school	RJ	Home		06 months
Orange	75	High school incomplete	RJ	Home		02 years
Brown	82	Complete primary education	PA	Home		01 year
Beige	45	Elementary school	RJ	Home		06 months

Note that the age of the clients varies from 30 to 82 years, with three clients are in their thirties. age group. The age of the person influences the how the disease alters their lives. Sexuality, the fact that the woman is in the reproductive phase, the possibility of mutilation (by hysterectomy, among other surgeries), the person's tolerance to pain, are all factors that must be taken into account.

The treatment time for the disease in question is long, with the shortest being three months and the longest two years among the clients interviewed. Some clients have been away from home since the start of therapy, while others travel daily for treatment. In addition to suffering from the disease, these clients have to deal with changes to their routine, given the length of cancer treatment.

Nurses' biographical data:

Codename	Time as a graduate	Oncology time	EC time	Titration
Pink	03 years	03 years	03 years	Specialization in Nursing Oncology
Green	02 years	02 months	02 months	In progress Specialization in Oncology Nursing
Fuchsia	27 years old	09 years	05 years	RxT Service Training
Grey	29 years old	06 years	05 years	In progress Specialization in Oncology Nursing
Brown	04 years	04 years	02 months	Specialization in Nursing Oncology
Golden	07 years	07 years	07 years	Specialization in Nursing Oncology

Table legend: EC - nursing consultation

The nurses' time since graduation ranges from two to twenty-nine years, and their experience with nursing consultations for the client in question ranges from two months to seven years. The nurses interviewed recognized the need for training, and all of them have different degrees for caring for oncology clients. Commitment to the profession, to care and to the nursing consultation activity emerged in all the statements, regardless of how long they had been trained. I believe that the need for efficient care, combined with scientific knowledge, leads to the concern mentioned.

Concrete categories of the lived experience that emerged from the clients' speeches, which indicated their motives:

Search for advisors

Clients seek nursing consultations in order to understand their current situation as cancer patients. Their natural attitude is to obtain knowledge about the disease and its treatment, in order to take care of themselves. The behavior of those who have the pathology in question is focused, from the moment of diagnosis, on the disease itself. The life of someone who finds out they have cancer is changed, regardless of how they approach this new phase in their life. This type of situation is defined by Schutz (1979, 2012) as a system of relevance, when we need to decide which elements should be transformed in our lives.

In the statements below, the clients express their desire to have information about the treatment itself, since the disease has come into their lives. Therefore, their intention is to find out more about the illness, so that they can take steps towards a new life situation. In this case, as a facilitator, it is up to the nurse to meet the educational needs of these clients, so that their full potential for coping with the illness can be harnessed, since their lifestyle habits can be modified:

"So we're looking for information. Because when you find out you're ill, you're left with no ground, you've been beaten down, you have no horizon, you're insecure, you don't know what to do. Then you need guidance, information about treatment. And that's what we have here... The nursing consultation is good because all this worry is in our heads, and the nurse explains about the treatment and how we should take care of ourselves, what we can and can't do. You become very sensitive, I even tried to read up on the disease to calm down more. When I came to the nurse's appointment, it was good because I wanted clarification, and I got it." Red

"The nursing consultation helped me, it explained a lot to me, I had doubts and I really wanted to ask some questions. I came with doubts, I came with fear, it's good that you give this consultation to guide us, because we come without knowing anything, the doctor explains but doesn't give details of the treatment." Yellow

"It was definitely worth it. I feel very tired, but I don't give in. And the nursing consultations help us face things and understand the treatment better." Orange

According to Schutz (1979, 2012), intersubjectivity is a situation shared by two or more people capable of communicating with each other. And if one understands the other's intention and corresponds to it, one meets their expectations. As in the testimonies below, in which the nursing consultation reveals itself as a form of care capable of meeting the clients' expectations, fulfilling its function, which is to seek solutions to the problems that arise. By meeting the needs of the clients, the nurse adapts the intention of the care to theirs, in a reciprocity of perspectives:

"I think coming to see you is good because we don't know how to take care of ourselves; I mean, when we start treatment we have a lot of doubts, the doctors can't tell us if we're going to be okay or not, if this disease is going to be cured... It was good for me because I cleared up my doubts... I think that if I hadn't come to the nurse's appointment it would have been even worse to face all this." Blue

"I wanted to know what it was about, I'd never been to this kind of appointment, I was curious. I knew I had to go through it, so I came. I liked it because I felt calmer with the explanations the nurses gave... This consultation with the nurses is good because it explains a lot and calms us down. I didn't know there was one, I liked it... We have doubts, we don't know if we can eat anything, if we can take medication... And here we learn about everything, until I understood everything correctly". Coral

"So, what I had in mind when I first came to the nurse's office were doubts about everything, because I came for treatment with no idea. I came from another hospital and here they taught me everything, so I have nothing to complain about, everything was excellent." Caramel

When clients refer to nursing, as Blue and Caramel did, they may be referring to a team of technicians or nurses. To clarify roles, I emphasize that nursing technicians provide low-complexity care, under the supervision of nurses, and that nurses plan and coordinate care, providing high-complexity care.

In our clients' search for care, I would emphasize the presence of the multidisciplinary team, with each professional acting according to their competence, joining forces to make the care happen. By referring clients to other specialties, we are strengthening this type of partnership. Guiding clients appropriately within the health system is the duty of all the teams involved, so that we can achieve humanized care. And in the process, we are all teaching and learning, clients and professionals alike.

Still reflecting on partnerships, I identified that in the process of caring, nurses must take into account the relationship between the person being cared for and their peers. In the following statement, I can see the importance of the family, inserted in the client's context. This is an example of educational action being extended to those who live with the client, which for Schutz's Phenomenology (1972, 2012) can be interpreted as "understanding the importance of the other's social network":

"So I went through the nursing consultation and I thought it was good. We come with questions in our heads and I thought the nurse clarified things and took away a bit of the fear, because we're a bit traumatized by it all, right? The consultation put me at ease... In the case of the consultation with the nurse, it reassured both me and my family, because when we get home, everyone wants to know how the treatment went, what's going on, what I did at the hospital that day, if the doctor said anything... So I think the nursing consultation is good because it clears up any doubts, I think that's what we come here for". Grafite

When seeking advice, the clients mentioned below reported a special concern for self-care. Just as their doubts are unique to each client, nursing advice must also take into account the uniqueness of each individual. The hope is that the nursing care provided during the consultation will help the clients to live with their cancer, making them as independent as their general state of health allows.

Understanding intentionality as acts of work in progress, directed towards the objects and objectives to be achieved (Schutz, 1979, 2012), the nurse's natural attitude when caring for the client in question should be to provide care that has meaning for her. After all, cancer is a devastating disease, with alarming statistics, often with a bleak prognosis (BRASIL, MS, INCA, 2012). Therefore, care planning for these clients should be carried out in a flexible manner, in order to take into account their biographical situation:

"I came with doubts to the nurse's appointment, I didn't know if I could take medication, if I could eat anything, if I could be around children, all that sort of thing. The nurses explained

everything that was being done to me, explained that brachytherapy is a complement to external radiotherapy, asked how I was getting on? The consultation with them was good because I wanted to know some things, I was afraid of doing something wrong and they explained everything to me... So it's very important for us to be clear about everything that's happening to us. That's the message I want to send you: we need to be clear about everything." Creme

"It's simple. If the nurse explains everything, the patient will know how to treat themselves. Sometimes patients do things wrong because they haven't been told. I'm one of those who does what I'm told; whatever I have to do for the good of my health, I do. That's why I think that what we have in mind when we come for a consultation is guidance... We need a lot of information to live with this disease. I eat well, I work well, I just have a bit of burning to urinate. We have a lot of doubts, one day is not the same as the next". Beige

"When I came to the nurse's appointment, I came to get advice, to find out about the treatment. In the other radiotherapy, we already know something, but the explanation here is more detailed, it explains things better, because the first doubt we have is how to take care of ourselves, if we can eat anything, if we can take medication, if we have to rest, these things." White

There is a common aspect in the clients' speeches: the importance of the educational process for them, when they mention seeking guidance. This should be done repeatedly throughout treatment, whenever necessary. The clients' situation regarding gynecological brachytherapy generates the natural attitude of trying to deal with the procedure in the best possible way for them.

The hope of a cure becomes a priority in these people's lives and all their efforts are directed towards this goal. This generates a typical pattern of behavior, which is that of wanting to be informed in order to experience the phase to come. Therefore, the need for a change in the behavior of these clients must be met according to the uniqueness of each of them, adapting the care proposal to these needs. This happens when the interests of the client and the nurse become mutual within the educational process.

This process is related to various practical issues, such as planning self-care at home and organizing the daily lives of these clients. In the interviews conducted for this study, the reasons that motivate clients to attend nursing appointments included fear, doubts in general, anxiety and a genuine need for clarification. If the world of human life changes with the onset of any illness, it is up to the nurse to accompany the sick person and their social network through this process of change, in order to live in the current reality.

Thus, I identify the value that guidance has for clients, and the educational process should be configured as nursing care within health units, and not just as an isolated activity, outside the context of care.

In this sense, teaching and learning is not just the reproduction of technical behaviors related to scientific procedures. It's teaching and learning how to think, act and behave appropriately in order to experience this life cycle, which is presented in the singularity of each individual, be they client or nurse. After all, the aim of the nursing consultation is to meet the needs of the human being, the main one being to live with quality of life.

Experiencing fear

The category arose because the feeling of fear can be very strong in people who find out they have cancer, varying between the subjects according to the meaning the disease has for each one. It can be represented by concern for the family, the relationship the disease has with death and/or the imminence of facing treatment, which is often long and traumatizing. This is due to the characteristics of the available therapies, which take a long time to respond to, involving surgery, chemotherapy, radiotherapy, bone marrow transplantation and other invasive, tiring and painful procedures.

In the following speeches, the clients reveal anguish about the uncertainty of the future, especially with regard to their children. They are also concerned about their social network, when they say it is distressing to be away from home, family and work. As they don't know what lies ahead, it's difficult for them to set priorities and decide on a course of action. Their lives are put on hold, only because of the importance of the illness. Faced with this situation, nurses must teach without pragmatism and learn with tolerance, giving their clients a voice, like the ones below:

"I have three little girls, my life is like this, o (she makes a sign with her hands that she's curled up). I had to leave my husband in Belem and come here with the girls, because I'd miss

them. Wow, our heads are in pain, this disease isn't easy". White

"For me, one thing that's difficult is being away from home, I have children and grandchildren, my daughter lives with me, I mean, I live with her... It's very bad to be away from my grandchildren. There are a lot of them, they get carried away, they make a mess and I miss that." Blue

"I have my children to bring up and I can't stand still, God forgive me, not knowing if I'm going to die or not. I'm sorry, but we have to be honest and really use our words. I just want to know if I'm going to be able to raise my children. Why am I saying all this? Simply because even in this phase of indecision about what's going to happen, you help us, you guide us. And that's very important. Bege

The prospect of finitude runs through the minds of clients and deserves special attention. Since the perception of death has a special meaning for each human being, nurses must be careful not to share their own values about dying. The professional must provide care from the perspective of phenomenological reduction, which happens when we leave our beliefs and opinions in abeyance in order to listen to what the other person is saying, without judging them (SCHUTZ, 1979, 2012). Therefore, the educational process must be based on what the client believes. The following accounts explain this:

"And when you find out you're ill, it's horrible! You think you're going to die soon, that nothing else is worthwhile... Then things settle down and you see that you're moving on, even if you don't want to." Brown

"I have my children to bring up and I can't stand still, God forgive me, not knowing if I'm going to die or not. I'm sorry, but we have to be honest and use the words. I just want to know if I'm going to be able to raise my children. Beige

"My neighbor, who was a good friend of mine, died of this disease and she was in too much pain, she complained a lot, she even died in my arms..." Lilas

During the process of becoming ill, the clients' biographical situation changes several times, depending on the stage of cancer treatment, and it is possible to compare their state of mind before and after treatment. The person diagnosed with cancer is removed from their world of life and placed in another, with which they have to live and establish new relevance, since their new priority is their health. According to Schutz's Sociological Phenomenology (1979, 2012), in this case it is necessary to consult the current stock of knowledge in order to make plans for the future. And solving (or not) the cancer issue takes priority over the original project, the one before the clinical diagnosis.

Even so, those who fall ill, although they have to live with new demands, don't abandon their previous knowledge because of their current state of health. The past is not erased. What changes is intentionality, which will be defined by how the individual faces the process of becoming ill. The following testimonies reflect the thoughts of those who have to move away from their world of life when facing cancer:

"I was really scared, because I'd never had anything sick... Then I started to feel pain and went to the health insurance doctor. I'm from the interior of São Paulo, and they told me to come here, and then I got some clarification: they told me what kind of tumor I had, and then I could start treatment. Look, I prefer to go back and forth every day, my city is right here. Even though I have to travel every day, I feel safe here... " Red

"You know what? At first it was all very, very horrible. I was angry, nervous, disgusted, because I was ill. There was that shock, and now I've come to terms with it, thank God, but when I found out I had this disease, wow! Now I'm fine, even more so because today is the last application, and I was dying to get out of here; I'm not from here, I'm from Minas Gerais, and you leave your house, your children, your grandchildren, your whole life on hold because of this treatment, how nice to go home!" (laughs). Yellow

"When I found out, I was calm, I mean, I was and I wasn't, because you get really worried, who doesn't when they're sick? Especially if you find out you have cancer, my God! Some days I'm calmer, some days I'm more worried... For me, one thing that's difficult is being away from home, I have children and grandchildren, my daughter lives with me, I mean, I live with her. I live far away from here, the journey is tiring, to come every day, I have to stay in a care home, and it's very bad to be away from my grandchildren. There are a lot of them, they get carried away, they make a mess and I miss that. And it's also bad to leave our home, to leave our things. I'm glad the treatment ended today, I'll be able to go home". Blue

"Now I just want to know if I'm going to get well. I want to go back to work, it can't go on like this, I only stopped because I got sick. Luckily, the service here is very good. The consultation with the nurse was good, because she talked to me, explained many things, but also asked about me, how I live, what I do for a living, and that was very good." Coral

The proximity of the end of treatment brings back the prospect of the future for the clients, who say they are relieved by this phase. For them, it is now possible to rethink their priorities, renew their intentions and plan their behavior for the future. Nursing care should also be geared towards the future, reinforcing with the client the importance of self-care and recalling what these should be, according to each client's needs. And, in this final phase, the nurse can reflect on the lessons learned with each client, when planning care for the next ones. The expectation of the end of treatment is described in the following statements:

"I'm still a bit nervous; I did my third application today and I'm dying to finish the treatment soon, I won't settle down until it's all over." Grena

"It's bad to leave your home, to leave your things. I'm glad the treatment ended today, I'll be able to go home." Blue

"Now, I just want to know if the treatment has worked; I'm dying to get it over with, to have the tests done soon to find out if I've been cured." Beige

"You explained it to me, it calmed me down a bit, but it's only after the treatment is over that we really feel relieved. It's good to know that it's over and that I don't have to have this treatment ever again!" Yellow

According to the testimonies, the fear of treatment has several aspects. Fear of the unknown can take on worrying dimensions and significantly affect the emotional side of clients if it is not managed or controlled. The feelings can be so distressing that they lead to the client giving up on treatment or the treatment becoming ineffective, as a result of the client not attending the health unit as she should, fulfilling all the stages of treatment.

In order to manage this unpleasant sensation (fear), the nurse can also count on the help of the multidisciplinary team, using psychology to deal with emotional issues, the doctor to prescribe drug therapy and social services to deal with legal issues, which are often priorities for the clients. And, as the nurse has access to all the members of the health team, he or she can also make sure that the client is being managed within the unit, helping the team in any way necessary.

In view of the above, it is important that all doubts are resolved, all questions exhausted, in the educational process. There is no such thing as a recurring question. A subject that hasn't been resolved is a subject that hasn't been explored as it should have been. Being afraid is a natural attitude for those with cancer. It's a feeling that will only diminish or cease to exist when everything related to it is handled properly.

If empathy is created during contact with the nurse, a helping relationship can be established between the nurse and the client, culminating in problem-solving. This characterizes the exchange that exists in the teaching and learning of each client and each nurse during the treatment process. The client learns and teaches how to manage her fears. And the nurse learns and teaches to understand the causes of these fears and to create possibilities for overcoming them.

Overcoming pain

A common element in the lives of cancer patients, pain can manifest itself in two ways: physically, as a result of the illness process, or emotionally, represented here by the psychological suffering caused by the pathology.

I understand that caring for people in pain, from the perspective of phenomenology, would mean getting to know the subject's experience of the event and what it means to them, with the aim of finding the best solution to the problem. To do this, there needs to be intersubjectivity, also defined by Schutz (1979, 2012) as the mutual understanding of the other's world, when we share experiences, in an intercommunication originating from a face-to-face relationship.

Physical pain occurs frequently in clients undergoing gynecological brachytherapy. When they report their experience of the event, it is up to the nurse to support them, using their technical skills to help them overcome the discomfort. The following reports reveal how common the occurrence of algias is in cancer patients. It is therefore desirable that all nurses working in this area receive training in pain control:

"I was really scared, because I'd never had anything painful; I'd go to the doctors and they'd even praise it. Then I started to feel pain and went to the health insurance doctor." Red
"You know, people said that this treatment was difficult, this last one, the brachytherapy,

but it's difficult! Daughter, it was horrible!... No one was prepared for that pain!!! Of course, without the nurse's consultation, it was going to be horrible. I felt all that pain, but I knew it was for my treatment. I just didn't know it would hurt so much". Yellow

The next story is an example of care aimed at the client's uniqueness, reflecting interaction with her. In this case, the treatment modality was modified to meet the needs of the client, who reported intense pain on the first attempt. In other words, the intentionality of the care was directed towards the client's motivation, which was not to feel physical pain:

"Since I was anesthetized today for the treatment, I'm going to stay here longer, because I had to be anesthetized and the other anesthetic for the next time can't be done until next week. I had to be anaesthetized, the first time they tried to do it without anaesthetic, you see, my God, it was torture!... Now I'm calmer, there's only one more to go. Cream

With regard to emotional distress, the clients report their anguish at the knowledge that they have an illness with an uncertain prognosis. They have to deal with worries about their family, the fear of death and the physical limitations imposed by the disease, just as they eventually have to deal with fear. As the feeling of suffering is unique to each person, I don't think it's appropriate to propose a single course of action for these clients.

In this way, it's essential to get to know each person's emotional state in order to feel what can be taught and what can be learned. And intersubjectivity appears in the nursing consultation. In this case, the educational process must remain open, depending on the intentions of each client. The following accounts reflect the emotional suffering of clients experiencing the treatment in question:

"Wow, our heads are in a lot of pain, this disease isn't easy. The fact that I had to leave my town really affected me. If there's anything we patients can teach you, it's that this treatment is very painful and very scary." White

"... When you find out you're ill, you're left with no ground, you're beaten down, you have no horizon, you're insecure, you don't know what to do." Red

"You know what? At first it was all very, very horrible. I was angry, nervous, disgusted, because I was ill. There was that shock, and now I've come to terms with it, thank God, but when I found out I had the disease, wow!" Yellow

According to the testimonies, I think that in order to overcome the painful process, regardless of its origin (physical or emotional), it is necessary to combine the technology of care with the uniqueness of each client. The nurse's intention should be to use scientific knowledge at the service of the human being, favoring their biographical situation.

Pain is known as an unpleasant sensory or emotional experience, and the nursing team is one of the most appropriate to assess this discomfort in clients, as well as their therapeutic response (BRASIL, MS, INCA, 2002b). Because it is unique, for each human being it has a meaning. Hence the fact that some people are more tolerant of algias than others. Therefore, culture, age and the extent of the disease itself must be taken into account when assessing pain in cancer patients.

The nurse assigned to relieve an algia crisis must be qualified to do so, if possible with training provided by the health unit. In order to manage this issue, I believe it is necessary for the professional to stick to the knowledge acquired through study and work, avoiding relying on value judgments or myths, but with the sensitivity to listen to each client in their individuality.

This means that, as it is a subjective fact, pain cannot be contested. And because it is a singular event, nurses must understand that **the pain the client says she feels is the pain she is feeling.** Therefore, in order to control it, the nurse's conduct and guidance must be based on the client's experience of the event.

In the case of a client who feels physical pain, the nurse should check that the client is taking pain medication. There are cases in which the Pain Clinic of the institution needs to follow up. The most effective therapeutic plan for controlling this discomfort is for the patient to spend twenty-four hours free from it, including sleeping and waking without pain (BRASIL, MS, INCA, 2002b). The priority in interacting with the client who feels pain is precisely to relieve it, avoiding manipulation before trying to solve the problem (ARAUJO, 2007).

With regard to emotional discomfort, it is essential to rely on the psychology team to manage the internal suffering caused by the pathology in question. When thinking of the client as a whole, nurses still need to be aware of the need for referrals to other members of the health team. Reflecting on the daily routine of teaching and learning in nursing consultations, I reiterate that the quality of what is taught or learned can be altered if both the teacher and the learner are in physical or emotional pain.

Three categories emerged from the speeches of the thirteen clients interviewed, based on their anxieties: **Seeking guidance, Experiencing fear and Overcoming pain.** According to Schutz (2012), the description of how a person experiences a phenomenon provides their lived type. Thus, it can be said that the **lived type** of the clients mentioned in this study is that of people who need guidance, feel afraid of the disease and the treatment and experience physical and emotional pain caused by the diagnosis and the procedures.

The clients' treatment routine provided me with data to draw up a profile of them, who have facts in common in their daily lives, constituting typical situations for those who experience the therapy in question. The subjects of the study are people undergoing long-term treatment, ranging from three months to two years. Some of the clients need to stay near the institutions in question in order to receive treatment, and are far from home and family because they live far away.

There are also clients who make short journeys to the place of treatment, but these are tiring because they are daily and because of the weakness that the disease causes. Many of them complain about the change in their routine, which is put on hold because of the therapy. This provides an opportunity to mess with their emotions, since when they are away from their normal routine, in the moments of rest between trips to the hospital, negative thoughts can arise about their biographical situation.

Schutz's system of relevance (1979, 2012) tells us that priorities are in our daily lives, appearing in a pure state or mixed together. These priorities have two origins: **intrinsic**, which are the result of the subject's interests and are chosen by him or her, and **imposed**, which are beyond the individual's control and are not chosen by him or her, generally translated into situations that arise in the human being's life and it is up to him or her to manage them.

Thus, for these clients, solving the problem of cancer takes priority over their previous life projects. This is when the imposed relevance becomes intrinsic, in other words, the clients didn't choose to get sick, but from the moment cancer came into their lives, the search for a cure became a priority in their lives.

Schutz (1979, 20012) states that the natural attitude is the stance taken by human beings in the face of facts and objectives. Since uncertainty about the future is a constant for the client undergoing gynecological brachytherapy, it is equally difficult for her to define a standard natural attitude towards cancer, since the pathology affects each person individually. It is up to the nurse to learn how this happens for each client and to help them experience the disease and the treatment.

Thinking about the individuality of the subjects of this study, it is gratifying to see that, with the practice of nursing consultation, the nurse becomes a reference point for them, in partnership with the other members of the hospital team.

I would also point out that there are clients with chronic illnesses, including cancer, who need to be stabilized in relation to these illnesses. The need for continuity of care and treatment is a reality. The nurse must make this continuity possible, since the client may be far away from the institution of origin.

In addition to suffering from the disease, the clients have to face difficult changes to their routine over a long period of time, given the length of cancer treatment. The anxieties described in the categories established do not depend on age or level of education; they are common to all, stemming from living with cancer. What changes is the way they present themselves and their intensity, which varies according to the uniqueness of each subject.

Concrete categories of the lived experience that emerged from the nurses' speeches, which indicated their motives:

The nurses reported that they considered educational activities to be important, mentioning that they should be tailored to the needs of the clients. For these professionals, clients should be taught self-care in a unique way, so that they have quality of life during and after treatment.

Attending to the singularity of the subjects in the treatment

The category arose from the nurses' experience that clients have their own individuality. After all, a client who is guided according to her basic needs tends to understand her illness and take care of herself in a satisfactory way, going through treatment with as few adverse events as possible.

According to Schutz (1979, 2012), when we direct our social action towards the motivations of our peers, we are adjusting intentions. And when we give our clients a voice, meeting their needs, we are creating opportunities for a relationship of exchange. Thus, we can always teach and learn from each other, and the teaching-learning process should be considered by nurses as care, since proper guidance leads to resolutions in nursing consultations.

The existence of the uniqueness of the clients, identified by the nurses interviewed, is present in the daily routine of care. This leads to different ways of conducting the nursing consultation, as described below; since, in the context of the institutions in question, clients can present themselves in the following ways:

- Crying for various reasons, such as fear of the disease and/or treatment, conflicts in the family or social life, among others. The nurse should offer this client a referral to the psychology service. This is necessary because psychological treatment is only beneficial if it is in the best interests of the person being treated. Therefore, before making the referral, the nurse should find out from the client if there are any restrictions on her part with regard to seeing a psychologist.

- Before he even sits down, he wonders if he can eat anything. She either shows progressive weight loss or mentions gastrointestinal disorders. The nurse's approach should be to refer this client to nutrition. Progressive weight loss is a worrying fact for cancer patients, as it can have an impact on their general condition and may even result in the need to interrupt treatment, which is not favorable for them.

- He mentions algia. It is clear that the guidelines run the risk of not being understood, given this condition. The nurse should try to solve the problem by following the client's pain medication regimen or referring her to the doctor or the Pain Clinic of the institution. The professional should be aware of the pain treatment protocol of the institution where she works, working with the multidisciplinary team to combat the problem. The client must also be told that the pain **is** to be treated. This is because it's common for cancer patients to consider that pain is part of their lives and that they need to get used to it.

- Even before the consultation begins, she asks questions about benefits or says that she doesn't have the financial resources to go to the institution as the treatment requires. She should be referred by the nurse to the Social Service, which will provide guidance to ensure that the cancer client's rights are guaranteed, as provided for in the MS's expande project. It is also important for the nurse to check whether there is any embarrassment on the part of the client due to her social condition.

- Adverse events resulting from the treatment appear on the skin. In cases of injury, the care administered during the nursing consultation is different for each client. Certain aspects need to be assessed, such as the extent and depth of the injury, as well as allergies. Expanding the interest to care for the mucous membranes of the urinary and intestinal tracts, it is important to know the pattern of the clients' physiological eliminations, asking about the existence of dysuria and/or tenesmus and finding out about their sexual activity.

In view of the above, the complexity of the teaching and learning process that takes place in the nursing consultation for the client in question is evident. And I emphasize that the way the client presents herself at the time of the consultation will influence the quality of what is taught and learned. Hence the importance of respecting the individuality of each human being. The speeches below illustrate how the nurses showed an interest in their clients' personal impressions about living with cancer:

"The teaching and learning that takes place in the nursing consultation is very important; we learn a lot from the patients. Each one has a different perception of the treatment, their experience is different. This enriches us and helps us plan care for these patients." Rosa

"I learn from each person's personal story. Some may have had skin lesions, others difficulty urinating; each one reacts in a different way. As a result, during brachytherapy I learn what they've been through before and what they're going through now, and this will help me direct the care for this treatment." Fucsia

"But what I really want is for the clients to ask any questions they have about the treatment. I also try to find out about their general condition, how they're feeling, how their life is in general during treatment." Ash

Empathy was cited by the nurses interviewed as an essential element in their relationship with clients. It should not be forgotten that cancer changes the lives of those who fall ill, so that the person has to learn to think in accordance with their new life experience. Therefore, the nurse must accompany the clients' reasoning about their feelings about the reality of having the disease. The reports recorded the emergence of a partnership between the parties involved in EC. After all, in the educational process there needs to be an exchange, as follows:

"Dal the importance of exchange, of teaching and learning: how are you going to talk about all this with the patient if you don't get along with her, don't listen to what she has to say, don't learn from her? I think this has something to do with quality of life after treatment." Rosa

"... We learn a lot from the patients' experiences, from everything related to their routine.

Especially because there are cases in which they (the patients) only tell their experiences to the nurses, and we recognize the importance, the value of this exchange." Green

"It's been gratifying to see our clients feel more at ease when they have their treatment. It's good to see that the consultation was of great benefit to both the nurses and the clients. This interaction helps us to know if we're on the right track." Ash

According to Schutz (1979, 2012), people tell facts and have their own wisdom, which comes from what they have experienced. Considering the author's words, I can see that in order to achieve the goals of the nursing consultation, care needs to be personalized for each client.

The fact is that the uniqueness of the human being can only be understood when you have direct contact with them. By taking an interest in the biography of each client with whom they come into contact, nurses get to know their universe. And the combination of these singularities will provide the typical (common) client, helping to build the model of care to be offered. This means that private interests can be in the same context as the interests of a group (SCHUTZ, 1979, 2012). Nurse Gray reinforces this reflection in her speech:

"Teaching and learning are very important. In some situations, the doubts that one client brings us may be the doubts of others. And with the knowledge that each client brings us, we can learn to act on the various points of doubt and solve the problems, or try to alleviate them. That's why I think it's important that all care comes from the client's needs."

The partnership mentioned by the nurses when dealing with their clients comes from a relationship of trust, typical of a face-to-face relationship, in which both subjects express their points of view in an intersubjective way. The nurse, knowing the clients' priorities and their intentions with regard to treatment, tends to adapt the care to what they have reported. However, reiterating Schutz's (2012) question, how is this mutual understanding possible; how can we attribute the correct meaning to what the other person is expressing? I agree with the author, who replies that in order to do this, we need to consider the strength of our fellow human beings' knowledge, respecting their privacy, as Nurse Brown said:

"You can't compare patient A with patient B, because the treatment may be the same, but the response will be different for each one. And by knowing the symptoms of one patient I can help

another, who knows? What I have in mind is this: you have to respect the baggage that each patient brings."

According to the above, it is clear that the nurse's intentional action must be developed by valuing the other and giving them a voice. Hence the importance of taking into account the background knowledge of the person being cared for. Nurse Fucsia also explains this reasoning by putting herself in the other person's shoes. There is empathy and intersubjectivity in her speech, even when she declares that she wouldn't want that experience for herself:

"Wow, of course we have a lot of involvement with patients, that's natural... I'm a woman too and I wouldn't want to be in their shoes... As the applications go on, they lose their fear and learn to trust us more. Then it becomes easier to look after them. I feel very involved with them, even more so because I'm a woman like them."

A practical example of the above, experienced by the author, was to puncture the client's vein where she said to puncture it, because there, in the place she was indicating, it was easier. In the practice of care, this means giving the other person a voice. Thus, the behavior of the person being cared for is being modified for their well-being and the behavior of the nurse is being modified according to the person of each client.

Valuing technical care

Naturally, due to the scientific knowledge acquired during their training, the nurses were concerned about the technicality of the nursing care provided. Even so, the professionals showed an interest in the clients' personal impressions of the treatment, according to the following reports:

"As for us nurses, we're focused on care, attentive to the patient's treatment process, wanting her not to have cancer anymore, but we can't forget that there's a personal life after this treatment." Rosa

"It ends up being an exchange. We explain what we know about the treatment, about how they should take care of themselves and they tell us how they are feeling about the treatment, they talk about their physical reactions too." Green

"So we explain the procedure, we explain how many people will be in the room, that there's an anesthesiologist, the anesthesia resident, the nursing staff, the radiotherapist, the X-ray

technician; everything is explained... We know how complicated it is for the patients"... Fuchsia

"... What I really want is for the clients to ask any questions they have about the treatment. I also try to find out about their general condition, how they are feeling, how their life is in general during the treatment. Apart from that, there's the follow-up that takes place during the applications." Ash

Currently, with the Systematization of Nursing Care in force, it is necessary for nurses to be concerned with the technology of care, since advances in this area are well advanced. Thus, the foundation of nursing care must be recorded so that knowledge of the techniques can be disseminated and the body of specific nursing knowledge can be consolidated.

Hence the Ministry of Health's recommendation, when it set up the Expande Project, that the training of nurses in the oncology sector is fundamental, determining that at least one professional should be a specialist in the oncology area, in order to plan care. By training nurses, they gain autonomy through scientific knowledge, with the power of decision to manage and develop care in an informed way, minimizing the suffering of clients.

However, according to what was said, it is possible to combine technical care with humanized care. For Schutz (1979, 2012), you can develop social action and put yourself in the other person's shoes at the same time. All you have to do is give your fellow human being a voice, while respecting their experience. In the speeches below, we can see how it is possible to carry out technical care and take an interest in the client's individuality. In this case, the care I'm referring to is guidance on vaginal dilation, a concern shown by the nurses:

"... We mustn't forget that there is personal life after this treatment. That even if the patient thinks she won't have a sexual partner anymore, she can find someone in the future. That sexual dysfunction is something serious." Rosa

"Some of them are more withdrawn, others already use the procedure as an excuse to leave out topics about their sex life. We end up getting into the feminine issue, so many of them don't want to talk about it. Then we remember the psychological issue and refer these clients to psychology, if they want to. It's all very difficult for them. Brown

"We teach care, we talk about preventing complications and we also try to find out a bit about the patients' lives, because it's no use just talking. We try to find out what life is like for them

at home, which can be difficult. They are advised to exercise vaginal dilation or have sex with their husband. But often the husband doesn't want to use a condom. Or he doesn't want to know if she's in pain, or he simply doesn't want to have sex. So he still insists on having sex. So she's embarrassed to talk about a delicate subject like this and we try to approach it in a lighter, easier way for her. We try to convey to the patient that she is the owner of her body, that she has to have autonomy and that her husband must respect her limits. Our patients are simple, many think they have to obey their husband. We end up learning this from them, because how are we going to change this situation? So we have to help them without demanding an attitude from them." Dourado

In view of the above, I would stress that the creation of a nursing care protocol must be done in such a way that nurses can adapt its foundations to the needs and reality of each client, respecting their uniqueness. As in the statement by Nurse Brown, in which it became clear that each client teaches something, indicating that care and the educational process must be tailored to the needs of the clients:

... "It's important that we adapt to patients. We have protocols, which of course we have to follow, but with exceptions. We end up not circumventing these protocols, but adapting them to each patient. I see that the more we work in this area, the more we learn from our clients. And the more we learn, the more lessons we can pass on to them".

By analyzing the above statements in the light of Schutz's Phenomenology (1979, 2012), nurses, by combining their concern for the individuality of their clients with scientific care, can match their clients' reasons for consulting with the professionals' reasons for caring, generating a reciprocity of perspectives. Finally, I agree with Amador, Gomes, Coutinho, Costa and Collet (2011) when they say that it is a challenge for nurses to learn to teach and learn, transforming knowledge into human conduct that is relevant to their professional practice, translated into care.

Nurses' interest in nursing consultations should be stimulated from the time they graduate. I believe it is essential to discuss the subject not only among undergraduates, but also among postgraduates and nurses in care practice. The challenge mentioned in the previous paragraph consists of teaching the practice of consultation and understanding that each nurse will have their own way of reflecting on this care. It can therefore be seen that the impact of teaching **and** practicing nursing consultations will be different for each nurse who consults and for each client who is consulted.

In view of the above, nurses need to recognize their competence in teaching and practicing nursing consultation, a form of care that cannot be delegated and carries with it the rationale that justifies the reasons for the professional's care.

The nurses' statements indicated two points in common, which gave rise to two categories: **Attending to the uniqueness of the subjects in treatment and Valuing technical care**. I dare to associate them with my own practice, since my care context is similar to that of the subjects in this study, which groups us together in the same **type of experience**, as explained below.

In the study, I identified nurses as professionals with the sensitivity to adapt individual care to technology. This allows for a flexible interpretation of the nursing actions recommended in the various protocols followed in health institutions through care, teaching, research and extension in the field of oncology. The testimonies of the professionals show that contact with the clients provides a face-to-face relationship, the result of valuing the baggage of knowledge that each client brings.

The nurses interviewed recognized the need for training, and all of them have a differentiated qualification for caring for oncology clients, which consists of taking the Oncology Nursing Specialization course, as recommended by the Ministry of Health. Commitment to the profession, to care and to the nursing consultation activity came up in all the statements, regardless of how long the professional had been trained. It is the nurses' interest in their training, in order to develop their social action.

The concern with technical care, combined with the client's individuality, justifies some of the actions that take place in the nurse's daily routine when caring for a client undergoing brachytherapy gynecology. It's a question of having a view that allows you to assess the client as a whole, looking for elements in her general condition that might indicate that the treatment should not be carried out at that time. This observation is important so that professionals can put themselves in the shoes of those being cared for, as this is the only way to achieve their goals in terms of excellent care.

Complementing the reflection in the previous paragraph, I would like to mention some aspects of care in this area, which can serve as examples: It is noticing if the client is eating correctly for her standards and is not showing significant weight loss. Evaluating the condition of the skin in the treatment area, looking for lesions and/or exudates. And ask if the client has any pain. Find out if the client has any other illnesses apart from cancer, if she needs to take continuous medication and if she is using it correctly. And to know the social condition in which the client lives. And to know the client's relationship with the disease and the treatment. And knowing how to assess the client so that she can be released after the procedure.

Finally, it's about understanding how the client relates to the institution and its various sectors, since treatment requires the interdisciplinary knowledge of the multi-professional team. In this way, the holistic care advocated in nurse training will be carried out, which should be based on satisfying the basic human needs of others.

The attention paid by some nurses to the vaginal dilation exercise deserves separate consideration, as it is considered one of the main tasks of care for the clients in question. Reflecting on their personal lives, it's easy to deduce that their priority is restoring their health. Therefore, it may be that the sexual issue is left in the background, as a personal relevance put on hold to attend to another relevance imposed by life. On the other hand, contrary to what was said earlier, sexual activity or vaginal dilation are indicated as a form of care. How can such activity be demanded of the client when this is not a priority for her?

It's a paradox, an installed situation that it's up to the nurse to help the client deal with. Psychology may be able to help, but the client needs to be willing to talk to the professional. The referral should be offered without insistence, leaving the client free to decide, since psychological treatment can be taboo for many people, due to the social prejudice that exists in relation to it.

In order to care for clients undergoing gynecological brachytherapy, I think it is necessary for nurses to set aside their personal impressions and put themselves in their shoes. This is a constant exercise. Professionals need to be aware of their clients' biographical situations and the meaning they attach to their lives, take into account that each client is unique and doesn't have to think like the others, and establish empathy with the client. By acting in this way, the chances are high that the product of the nurse's actions will be the satisfaction of the client's needs, in a reciprocity of intentions.

8. FINAL CONSIDERATIONS

In this chapter, I present my final suggestions for concluding this study, reiterating that reflection on the subject should continue through further research.

FINAL CONSIDERATIONS

According to cancer statistics from around the world, the political, social and human impact that this disease has on the lives of people and their families can be seen in the need for early diagnosis and immediate treatment. For this reason, the Expande Project was created in 2001, with the aim of distributing oncology care centers throughout the country, as well as promoting the training of professionals. And, as the population needs to have easy access to the health system, legislation was introduced in November 2012 which recommends that the time between clinical diagnosis and the start of treatment should be up to sixty days.

It all started with a situational map of Brazil, verifying the specific demands of the regions, according to the statistics of the disease in each location and analyzing the resources for clinical diagnosis. Hence the need to train the health team to work in oncology, generating specialization and residency courses in the various areas of the sector.

The educational actions to be carried out in this area include permanent education in institutions and actions aimed at clients, who are becoming more demanding in their search for care in health units and more receptive to the guidance they receive. Oncology training should also be extended to professionals from other areas, so that they can identify problems and make the appropriate referrals whenever necessary. The discussion of technical care among the multidisciplinary team becomes relevant when planning care for clients, and every specialty should maintain a training program for professionals from other areas.

It is clear that teaching and learning are not simple tasks. For this to happen, the intentions of those who teach and those who learn must be in harmony.

It is necessary to respect each other's potential, whether they have limitations or not, recognizing that every pace of learning is valid, as long as the goal between the subjects is achieved. All those involved in this process need to recognize that they have as much to teach as they do to learn, without vanity. And the process is changeable, because the experience of human beings changes, as do their priorities (relevance). This makes it possible to live with different situations.

I identified, through the practice of care, that the gynecological brachytherapy procedure takes place in the two settings of the study, based on interdisciplinarity, in which professionals from different areas work together to make the treatment happen. Teaching and learning did not only take place from the nurse to the client and from the client to the nurse. It happened equally between the professionals involved. As a result of this exchange of experiences, all the teams are caring for **and** treating the clients simultaneously, in all their different modalities. These teams include nurses, doctors, physios, psychologists, social workers, nutritionists, administrative secretaries and cleaners.

Therefore, the situation described below reinforces the value of educational action for clients, confirming their adherence to treatment: *two of the clients' relatives made a point of expressing their intentions with regard to the nursing consultation, even though they were aware that they would not be included as research subjects. Both pointed out that the consultation enlightens them as well, providing support for the care of their family member, and briefly described how they carry out this care. They recognized the importance of the nurse's work and insisted on answering the same questions as the clients, even though they knew that their statements would not be recorded as the focus of the study.*

As a result, we can see how beneficial it can be for clients to receive care from nurses throughout treatment and during nursing consultations, including clients and their caregivers, enabling quality of life during this phase. This experience has revealed a clientele that looks to the nurse as a reference professional when seeking guidance on how to deal with treatment.

Moreover, the practice of care shows us that care, when not carried out or carried out inefficiently, can influence the general state of the client and even the lives of family members.

I wouldn't dare suggest a specific approach for clients undergoing gynecological brachytherapy, since each client is unique and each nurse has their own approach to care. In addition, each institution has its own reality. Therefore, what I propose is a possibility of care, as described in chapters three and four of this thesis, which must be adapted to the needs of each situation.

However, some criteria can be adopted when structuring care for the client in question:

- Nursing consultations should be instituted for this client before treatment, as official care. Institutions need to pay attention to teaching and practicing this type of care, drawing up rules and routines for it.

- The nurse has to be in agreement and in tune with the other members of the multidisciplinary team, so that the procedure takes place properly, efficiently, effectively and safely for the client.

- The nurse's assistance should take place throughout the client's treatment phase, after which he or she should maintain the bond and the client should be advised to return even without an appointment.

- It is important for nurses to care for, treat and defend their clients' rights. Your knowledge as a professional in the field of oncology allows you to do this.

Given the above, I reiterate the value of learning to teach and learning to think about the experiences between clients and nurses in the nursing consultation for gynecological brachytherapy treatment. The teaching and learning that emerges helps us to understand that each client has a different level of understanding and that it is important to personalize this teaching in order to care for the other.

The need to carry out the study arose from the practice of care, giving me a new look at nursing care after this journey. The description of how the nursing consultation is carried out for clients undergoing gynecological brachytherapy at the HUCFF originated initially in informal meetings with the clients, giving voice to the subject for whom the care is carried out. It was later consolidated with this thesis. As the first fruit of this work, I can foresee a review of the protocols of the HUCFF Radiotherapy Service, scheduled for the semester following the conclusion of this work.

By disseminating the nurse's way of caring at the HUCFF Radiotherapy Service, I hope to provide readers with what has been learned along this journey. This study is intended for the clients who face gynecological brachytherapy treatment, the nurses who care for them and the family members who, although they were not part of it, were present, sharing in this teaching and learning. Without the latter, it would not have been possible to stimulate interest in enduring the difficult moments of ignorance, pain, loneliness, coping and even joy for each of these clients.

In this sense, this thesis does not come to an end, but rather awakens the possibility of further work that includes the family, emphasizing the value of the partnership between human beings in the intentional action of nursing consultation.

REFERENCES

AMADOR, DD; GOMES, IP; COUTINHO, SED; COSTA, TNA; COLLET, N. Concepción dos enfermeiros acerca da capacitación no cuidado a crianga com cancer. **Texto contexto - enferm,** Florianopolis, 2011; v. 20 n°1 jan/mar

ARAUJO, CRG. **The meaning of the nursing consultation in the radiotherapy sector of the Clementino Fraga Filho University Hospital, as approached by clients and caregivers.** 2007. 123 f. Dissertation (Master's in Nursing) - Anna Nery School of Nursing, UFRJ, Rio de Janeiro, 2007

ARAUJO, CRG; ROSAS, AMMTF. The role of the nursing team in the radiotherapy sector: a contribution to the multidisciplinary team. **Revista Brasileira de Cancerologia,** RJ, 2008; 54: 231-37, n3

ARAUJO, CRG; ROSAS, AMMTF. The nursing consultation for clients and their caregivers in the radiotherapy sector of the University Hospital. **Rev. Enferm. UERJ,** RJ, 2008; 16(3): 364-9

ARAUJO, CRG. **Systematization of the nursing consultation for tracheostomized clients in the radiotherapy sector.** Monograph (Specialization in Oncology Nursing) - National Cancer Institute and Anna Nery Nursing School, UFRJ, Rio de Janeiro, 2002

ASA (American Society of Anesthesiologists). **Guidelines for ambulatory anesthesia and surgery.** Available at: <http://www.asahq.org/publicationsand   services/standards/04.pdf> Accessed on September 12, 2009

AYOUB, Andrea (Org.). **Planning care in oncology nursing.** Sao Paulo, Lemar, 2000. 292 p.

BARBOSA, MARS; TEIXEIRA, NZF; PEREIRA, WR. Nursing consultation - a dialog between technical and popular health knowledge. **Acta Paul. Enf.,** Cuiaba, 2007; 20(02): 226-9

BASTABLE, S (Org.). **The nurse as educator.** Porto Alegre: Artmed, 2010

BORGES, SC. **The vaginal dilation exercise after high-dose-rate brachytherapy: women's experiences.** 2003. 154 f. Dissertation (Master's in Nursing) - Anna Nery School of Nursing, UFRJ, Rio de Janeiro, 2003

BORK, AMT. **Evidence-based nursing.** Rio de Janeiro: Editora Guanabara Koogan, 2005

BRAZIL. Federal Nursing Council. **Cofen - Resolutions and legislation.** Available at: <http://www.portalcofen.gov.br> Accessed in October 2009

BRAZIL. Ministry of Health. National Cancer Institute. Standardization committee **Radiotherapy and you.** Rio de Janeiro: INCA, 2002a

BRAZIL. Ministry of Health. National Cancer Institute. **A^oes de enfermagem para o cancer control:** uma proposta de integragao ensino-servigo. 3ª ed. Rio de Janeiro: INCA, 2008

BRAZIL. Ministry of Health. National Cancer Institute. **Cancer palliative care;** pain control. Rio de Janeiro: INCA, 2002b

BRAZIL. Ministry of Health. **Standards for outpatient anesthesia.** Available at: <http://www.portaria MS n°44/ GM, de **10/01/2OO1**> Accessed in October 2009

BRAZIL, Ministry of Health. **Expande Project.** Available at : <http ://www. saude. gov.br> Ordinance 3.535 of 1998. Accessed in October 2011

BRAZIL. Ministry of Health. National Cancer Institute. **Radiotherapy and High Dose Rate Brachytherapy.** Available at: <http://www.radioterapia.org.br/radiofra.htm> Accessed in September 2009

BRAZIL. Ministry of Health. **Systematization of nursing care.** Available at : <http://www.saude.gov.br> Accessed October 2009

BRAZIL. Ministry of Health. National Cancer Institute. <www.inca.gov.br> Accessed from June to November 2012

CAPALBO, C. **Phenomenology and human sciences.** Sao Paulo: Editora Iddias e letras, 2008

CAPALBO, C. **Metodologia das ciencias sociais:** ªfenomenologia de Alfred Schutz. 2.ª ed. Londrina: Ed. UEL, 1998

CARVALHO, A.S. **Metodologia da Entrevista:** uma abordagem fenomenologica. 27 ed. Rio de Janeiro: Agir, 1991

DENARDI, UA (Org.) **Nursing in radiotherapy.** Sao Paulo: Lemar, 2008

DIEGUES, SRS; PIRES, AMT. The role of nurses in radiotherapy. **Revista Brasileira de Cancerologia,** RJ, 1997; 43(4): 251-5, Oct/Dec

FEUO, AM; SCHWARTZ, E; JARDIM, VMR; LINCK, C; ZILLMER, JGV; LANGE, C. O papel da família sob a otica da mulher acometida por cancro de mama. **Cienc. cuid. saude,** Pelotas, 2009; 8 (supl): 79-84 dec

FIGUEIREDO, NMA; LEITE, JL; MACHADO, WCA; MOREIRA, MC; TONINI, T. (Org.) **Enfermagem Oncologica** - conceitos e praticas. Sao Paulo: Yendis, 2009

GATES, R; FINK, R (Org.). **Secrets in oncology nursing** - necessary answers to everyday life. 3ª ed. Porto Alegre: Artmed, 2009

LOPES, MJM; SIVEIRA, DT; FERREIRA, SRS. Education and health in chronic degenerative diseases and the promotion of quality of life: an experience report. **Estud. interdiscip. envelhec.,** Porto Alegre, 1999; v.2 p.121-30

MACHADO, MMT; LEITAO, GCM; HOLANDA, FUX. The concept of communicative action: a contribution to nursing consultation. **Rev. Latino-Am. Enfermagem,** Ribeirao Preto, 2005; v.13 n°5 sep/out

MACHADO, SM; SAWADA, NO. Quality of life assessment of cancer patients undergoing adjuvant chemotherapy. **Texto contexto - enferm,** Florianopolis, 2008; v. 17 nº4 oct/dez

MARTINS, J & BICUDO, M A. **Studies on Existentialism, Phenomenology and Education.** Sao Paulo: Martins, 1983. 80 p

MICOZZI, T. in lecture on Scientific Production in Nursing, at the **2nd International Meeting: Knowledge Production and Nursing Research Centers,** EEAN/ UFRJ, October 16, 2008.

MOHALLEM, AGC; RODRIGUES, AB (Org.). **Enfermagem Oncologica.** Sao Paulo: Manole, 2007

MUNIZ, RM; ZAGO, MMF; SCHWARTZ, E. The webs of cancer survival: with life again. **Texto contexto - enferm,** Florianopolis, 2009; v. 18 nº1 jan/mar

PANOBIANCO, MS; PIMENTEL, AV; ALMEIDA, AM; OLIVEIRA, ISB. Women with advanced diagnosis of cervical cancer: coping with the disease and treatment. **Revista Brasileira de Cancerologia,** RJ, 2012; 58(3) 517-523

PELLIZZON, Antonio (Org.). **Routines and procedures in radiotherapy.** 3ª ed. Sao Paulo: Lemar, 2008

POLIT, DF.; BECK, CT ; HUNGLER, BP. **Fundamentals of Nursing Research** - methods, evaluation and utilization. 5th ed. Sao Paulo: Artmed, 2004

POPIM, RC; BOEMER, MR. Caring in oncology from Alfred Schutz's perspective. **Revista Latino-Americana de Enfermagem,** Ribeirao Preto, 2005; v.13, nº5

ROSA, MTS; SALES, CA. Experiences of women undergoing brachytherapy: existential understanding. **Rev. Eletr. Enf.;** Goiania, 2008; 10(4): 990-1003

ROSAS, AMMTF. **The nursing consultation in the health unit:** a comprehensive analysis from the nurses' perspective. 1998. 95 f. Dissertation (Master's in Nursing) - Anna Nery School of Nursing, UFRJ, Rio de Janeiro, 1998

ROSAS, AMMTF. **Teaching the care activity - nursing consultation:** the typical of intentional action. 2003. 180 f Thesis (Doctorate in Nursing) - Anna Nery Nursing School, UFRJ, Rio de Janeiro, 2003

SANTANA, GO. **Educational practice in nursing consultations:** a dialogic approach to children's learning. 2002. Dissertation (Master's in Nursing) - Anna Nery School of Nursing, UFRJ, Rio de Janeiro, 2002

SANTOS, MD. **Teaching-learning strategies in nurse training:** the ideology that permeates public health nursing teaching at Severino Sombra University. 2003. Dissertation (Master's in Nursing) - Anna Nery School of Nursing, UFRJ, Rio de Janeiro, 2003

SANTOS, R. **O significado da agao educativa consulta de enfermagem no ambulatorio de quimioterapia infantil:** perspectiva dos familiares. 2009. 110 f Dissertation (Master's in Nursing) - Anna Nery School of Nursing, UFRJ, Rio de Janeiro, 2009

SARAIVA, RJ. **The nursing consultation with the elderly adult:** a comprehensive analysis as a contribution to teaching. 2011. Dissertation (Master's in Nursing) - Anna Nery School of Nursing, UFRJ, Rio de Janeiro, 2011

SCHUTZ, A. **Collected Papers 1 - The Problem of Social Reality.** Netherlands: Martins Nijhoff, The Hague, 1962.

SCHUTZ, A. **Phenomenology and social relations.** Org. H.R. Wagner. Rio de Janeiro: Zahar, 1979

SCHUTZ, A. **On phenomenology and social relations.** Org. H.R. Wagner. Petropolis, RJ: Vozes, 2012

SILVA, MP; GANNUNY, C; AIELLO, NA; HIGINIO, MAR; FERREIRA, ON; OLIVEIRA, MMF. Evaluation methods for post-radiotherapy vaginal stenosis. **Revista Brasileira de Cancerologia,** RJ, 2010; 56(1): 71-83

UICC (International Union Against Cancer). **Manual of Clinical Oncology.** Sao Paulo: Editora FOSP, 2006

TREZZA, MCSF. **Contributing to the possibilities of liberation through illness for another way of living:** a theoretical model representing the experience of people who have had cancer. 2002. Thesis (Doctorate in Nursing) - Anna Nery School of Nursing, UFRJ, Rio de Janeiro, 2002

VANZELLI, TL; CARVALHO, FS; LIMA, SR. Barretos Cancer Hospital. **Norms and Routines of the Radiotherapy Service** - gynecological brachytherapy, 2009

VANZIN, Arlete; NERY, Maria Helena. **Nursing consultation:** a social necessity? 2ª ed. Porto Alegre: R M & L, 2000

VIANA, LO; SANTOS, MSS; VALENTE, GS; ROSAS, AMMTF; SANTOS, NMP; SILVA, CMSLMD. **Nursing Education and Health Research Center (NUPESENF - EEAN/UFRJ):** creation and consolidation of research lines, 2009

APENDICES

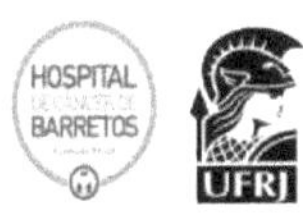

INFORMED CONSENT FORM

Version for nurses:

Dear nurse:
I am developing a work entitled **"TEACHING AND LEARNING IN NURSING CONSULTATION BETWEEN CLIENTS AND NURSES IN THE TREATMENT BY GYNECOLOGICAL BRACHITERAPY: A PHENOMENOLOGICAL APPROACH".** This is a doctoral thesis being carried out at the Anna Nery School of Nursing at the Federal University of Rio de Janeiro. My objectives are to identify the expectations of clients and nurses in teaching and learning in the nursing consultation in gynecological brachytherapy treatment and to discuss the links between the intentions expressed by nurses and clients about teaching and learning in the nursing consultation in gynecological brachytherapy treatment. I believe that the educational process that takes place during nursing consultations enlightens both clients and nurses, helping clients to optimize their self-care and nurses to plan their care. The aim is to find out what clients expect from their treatment and what it means for nurses to provide care through nursing consultations.

Your collaboration will be important in the sense that, based on the answers obtained, it will be possible to adapt nursing care to the clients, according to the needs pointed out by everyone. In other words, your help will help us to improve nursing care in the sector. This is the benefit of the study.

If you agree to take part, I will conduct a recorded interview. You are guaranteed the freedom not to want to take part in this work or to withdraw your consent at any time. You are also guaranteed the right to refuse to answer any question that may cause embarrassment of any kind. The interviews will be recorded using a voice recorder (with MP4 software) and the interviewees will have the right to anonymity, i.e. they will not be identified and their names will be replaced by colored names. The recordings will be erased from the device after five years.

The interview will take place according to your availability; the day, time and place will be scheduled according to your schedule.

The information obtained from each interviewee will be analyzed together with the information from the other interviewees, while maintaining due confidentiality. The data collected will only be used for this research, and the researcher is entirely responsible for its safekeeping.

No medical records or any other documents of the client interviewed will be used. No images of people will be used. Participants will have the right to know the progress of the research at any time. There will be no personal expenses for those who wish to participate, nor will there be any financial compensation related to the research, since this work is of low cost. There will be no risk of any kind (physical, mental or any other). The questions I will ask are:

- Tell us how you plan and carry out the nursing consultation in brachytherapy treatment.
- What do you have in mind when you teach and learn from your clients in the nursing consultation during brachytherapy treatment?
- What does it mean for you to teach and learn from clients during CE in brachytherapy treatment?

The interviewees will also be asked about some biographical data, such as: degree (courses

95

taken after graduation), age, time since graduation and how long they have been working in brachytherapy, performing the CE activity.

At any stage of the study, participants will have access to the researcher by telephone: nurse Claudia: 25622136 (radiotherapy), or by e-mail: .clauregingomes@hotmail.com

Contact with the study supervisor: Prof. Dr Ann Mary Machado Tinoco Feitosa Rosas: e-mail: annmaryrosas@gmail.comT 22930528 -EEAN/UFRJ

HUCFF/UFRJ Ethics Committee: telephone: 25622480 e-mail: cep@hucff.ufrj.brEnderego: R. Prof. Rodolpho Rocco, 255, Ilha do Fundao, 1°andar., sala 01D-46.

Barretos Cancer Hospital Ethics Committee:cep@hcancerbarretos.com.br telephone: 33216600 r. 6894.

The results of the research will be known at a public defense (presentation), scheduled for November 2012. Thank you very much.

Nurse Claudia Regina Gomes de Araujo

I believe I have been sufficiently informed about the above-mentioned work and have read the request for permission to take part.

I have spoken to nurse Claudia Regina Gomes de Araujo about my decision to take part in this study. I am aware that only one recorded (voice) interview will be carried out and that I will be guaranteed anonymity and ongoing clarification. I am also aware that my participation is free of charge, both for me and for the researcher. It is clear to me that the research will not interfere with my activities. I am also aware that the study is risk-free. I voluntarily agree to take part in the study and can withdraw my consent at any time if I wish. I am aware that the researcher and I must initial the pages of this Informed Consent Form. It will be drawn up in two copies, one for the study subject and one for the researcher.

Name of interviewee	Signature

Name of researcher	Signature

Witness	Signature

Date_________________/___/____

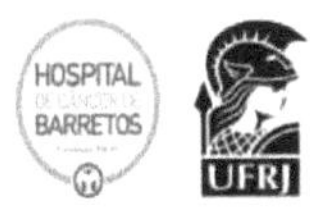

INFORMED CONSENT FORM

Version for customers:

Dear customer:
I am developing a work entitled **"TEACHING AND LEARNING IN NURSING CONSULTATION BETWEEN CLIENTS AND NURSES IN THE TREATMENT BY GYNECOLOGICAL BRACHITERAPY: A PHENOMENOLOGICAL APPROACH"**. This is a doctoral thesis being carried out at the Anna Nery School of Nursing at the Federal University of Rio de Janeiro. My objectives are to identify the expectations of clients and nurses in teaching and learning in the nursing consultation in gynecological brachytherapy treatment and to discuss the links between the intentions expressed by nurses and clients about teaching and learning in the nursing consultation in gynecological brachytherapy treatment. I believe that the exchange of information that takes place during nursing consultations enlightens both clients and nurses, helping clients to take better care of themselves and nurses to plan their care. The aim was to get to know the clients' expectations of the treatment and what it means for nurses to provide care through nursing consultations.

Your collaboration will be important in the sense that, based on the answers obtained, it will be possible to adapt nursing care to the clients, according to the needs pointed out by everyone. In other words, your help will help us to improve nursing care in the sector. This is the benefit of the study.

If you agree to take part, I will conduct a recorded interview. You are guaranteed the freedom not to want to take part in this work or to withdraw your consent at any time. You are also guaranteed the right to refuse to answer any question that may cause embarrassment of any kind. The interviews will be recorded using a voice recorder (with MP4 software) and the interviewees will have the right to anonymity, i.e. they will not be identified and their names will be replaced by colored names. The recordings will be erased from the device after five years.

The interview will take place according to your availability; the day, time and place will be scheduled according to your wishes.

The information obtained from each interviewee will be analyzed together with the information from the other interviewees, while maintaining due confidentiality. Their answers will only be used for this research and will be kept under the researcher's full responsibility.

No medical records or any other documents of yours will be used. We will not use images of people. You will have the right to know the progress of the research at any time. There will be no personal expenses for those who wish to participate, nor will there be any financial compensation related to the research, since the work is low cost. There will be no risk of any kind (physical, mental or any other). The questions I will ask are:
- What do you have in mind when it comes to EC brachytherapy?
- How do you experience teaching and learning in brachytherapy treatment?
- Tell us what it has meant to you to teach and learn with EC in brachytherapy treatment.

The interviewees will also be asked about some data, such as: length of cancer treatment, age, education, profession, place of birth and whether they have ever suffered from a gynecological disease.

At any stage of the study, participants will have access to the researcher by telephone: nurse Claudia: 25622136 (radiotherapy), or by e-mail: .clauregingomes@hotmail.com

Contact with the study supervisor: Prof. Dr Ann Mary Machado Tinoco Feitosa Rosas: e-mail: annmaryrosas@gmail.comT 22930528 -EEAN/UFRJ

HUCFF/UFRJ Ethics Committee: telephone: 25622480 e-mail: cep@hucff.ufrj.brAddress: R. Prof. Rodolpho Rocco, 255, Ilha do Fundao, 1°andar., sala 01D-46.

Barretos Cancer Hospital Ethics Committee:cep@hcancerbarretos.com.br telephone: 33216600 r. 6894.

The results of the research will be known at a public defense (presentation), scheduled for November 2012. Thank you very much.

Nurse Claudia Regina Gomes de Araujo

I believe I have been sufficiently informed about the aforementioned work and have read the request for permission to take part in it.

I have spoken to nurse Claudia Regina Gomes de Araujo about my decision to take part in this study. I am aware that only one recorded interview (voice) will be carried out and that I will be guaranteed anonymity (secrecy) and ongoing clarification. I also understand that my participation is free of charge, both for me and for the researcher. It is clear to me that the research will not interfere with my treatment. I am also aware that the study is risk-free. I voluntarily agree to take part in the study and can withdraw my consent at any time if I wish. I am aware that both the researcher and I must initial the pages of this Informed Consent Form. It will be drawn up in two copies, one for the study subject and one for the researcher.

Name of interviewee	Signature

Researcher's name	Signature

Witness	Signature

Date________________/ ____ / ____

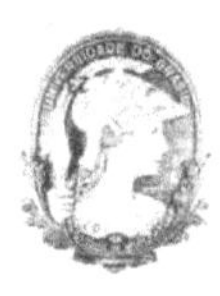

UNIVERSIDADE FEDERAL DO RIO DE JANEIRO
CENTRO DE CIÊNCIAS DA SAÚDE
ESCOLA DE ENFERMAGEM ANNA NERY
COORDENAÇÃO GERAL DE PÓS-GRADUAÇÃO E PESQUISA

Rio de Janeiro, 09 de setembro de 2011

Ao Hospital Universitário Clementino Fraga Filho

CARTA DE APRESENTAÇÃO

Apraz-nos apresentar a aluna **CLÁUDIA REGINA GOMES DE ARAÚJO**, registro UFRJ nº **110004536** regularmente matriculada no Curso de Doutorado em Enfermagem da EEAN da Universidade Federal do Rio de Janeiro.

Outrossim, vimos solicitar autorização para que o supra referido, possa coletar dados com a finalidade de desenvolver sua Tese de Doutorado.

Atenciosamente,

Jorge Anselmo
Secretário dos Cursos de
Pós-Grad./EEAN/UFRJ
Matr 0360956

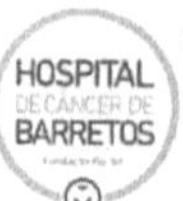

Comitê de Ética em Pesquisa
CEP

Para: Cláudia Regina Gomes de Araújo

De: Dr. Rafael Darahem de Souza Coelho
Vice- Coordenador do Comitê de Ética em Pesquisa

Data: 18/11/2011

Projeto de Pesquisa: **551/2011**

Prezado (a) Senhor (a),

Vimos, por meio desta, informar que o Comitê de Ética em Pesquisa da Fundação Pio XII – Hospital de Câncer de Barretos analisou as respostas às pendências do projeto de pesquisa **551/2011 "O ensinar e aprender na consulta de enfermagem entre clientes e enfermeiras no tratamento por braquiterapia ginecologica: uma abordagem fenomenológica"**, decidindo que o mesmo encontra-se: ***"Aprovado".***

Solicitamos que sejam encaminhados ao CEP, <u>relatórios semestrais e final</u>, bem como passíveis emendas e novos termos de consentimento livre e esclarecido, notifique qualquer evento adverso sério ocorrido no centro e novas informações sobre a segurança do estudo a fim de se fazer o devido acompanhamento.

Atenciosamente,

Dr. Rafael Darahem de Souza Coelho
Vice-Coordenador do Comitê de Ética em Pesquisa
Hospital de Câncer de Barretos

100

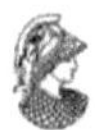

UNIVERSIDADE FEDERAL DO RIO DE JANEIRO
Hospital Universitário Clementino Fraga Filho
Faculdade de Medicina
Comitê de Ética em Pesquisa - CEP

CEP - MEMO – n.º 1142/11   Rio de Janeiro, 30 de dezembro de 2011.

Do: Coordenador do CEP

A (o): Sr. (a) Pesquisador (a): Cláudia Regina Gomes de Araujo

Assunto: Parecer sobre projeto de pesquisa.

Sr. (a) Pesquisador (a),

Informo a V. S.a. que o CEP constituído nos Termos da Resolução n.º 196/96 do Conselho Nacional de Saúde e, devidamente registrado na Comissão Nacional de Ética em Pesquisa, recebeu, analisou e emitiu parecer sobre toda documentação entregue em formato digital incluindo seu respectivo protocolo de pesquisa, conforme abaixo discriminado:

Protocolo de Pesquisa: 127/11 - CEP

Título: "O ensinar e aprender na consulta de enfermagem entre clientes e enfermeiras no tratamento por braquiterapia ginecológica: uma abordagem fenomenológica"

Pesquisador (a) responsável: Cláudia Regina Gomes de Araujo

Data de apreciação do parecer: 22/12/2011

Parecer: "APROVADO"

Informo ainda, que V. Sa. deverá apresentar relatório semestral, previsto para 22/06/2012, anual e/ou relatório final para este Comitê acompanhar o desenvolvimento do projeto. (item VII 13.d, da Resolução n. º 196/96 – CNS/MS).

Atenciosamente,

Prof. Carlos Alberto Guimarães
Coordenador do CEP

101

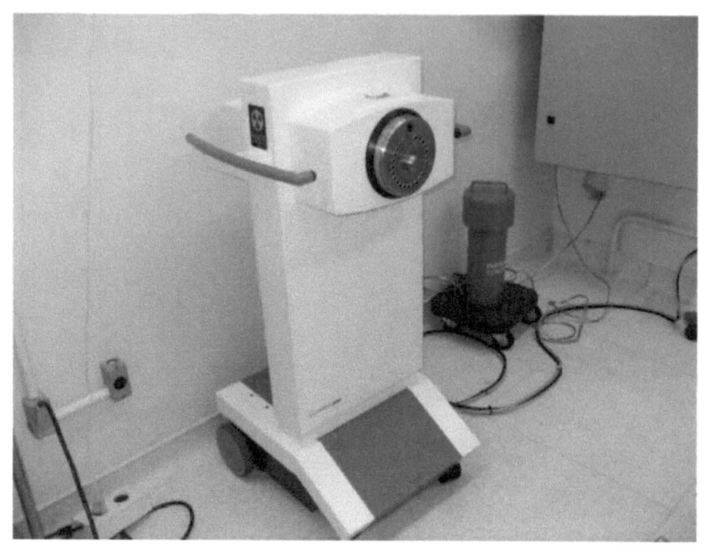

IRIDIUM SOURCE[192]

COLLECTION OF NURSE CLAUDIA R. G. ARAUJO

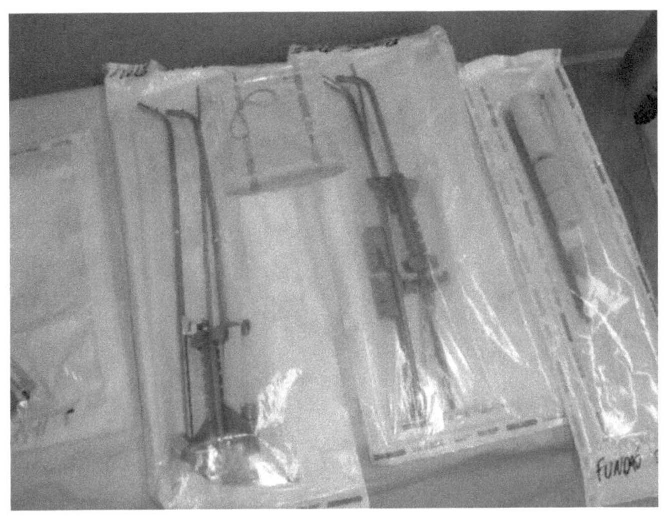

APPLICANTS

COLLECTION OF NURSE CLAUDIA R. G. ARAUJO

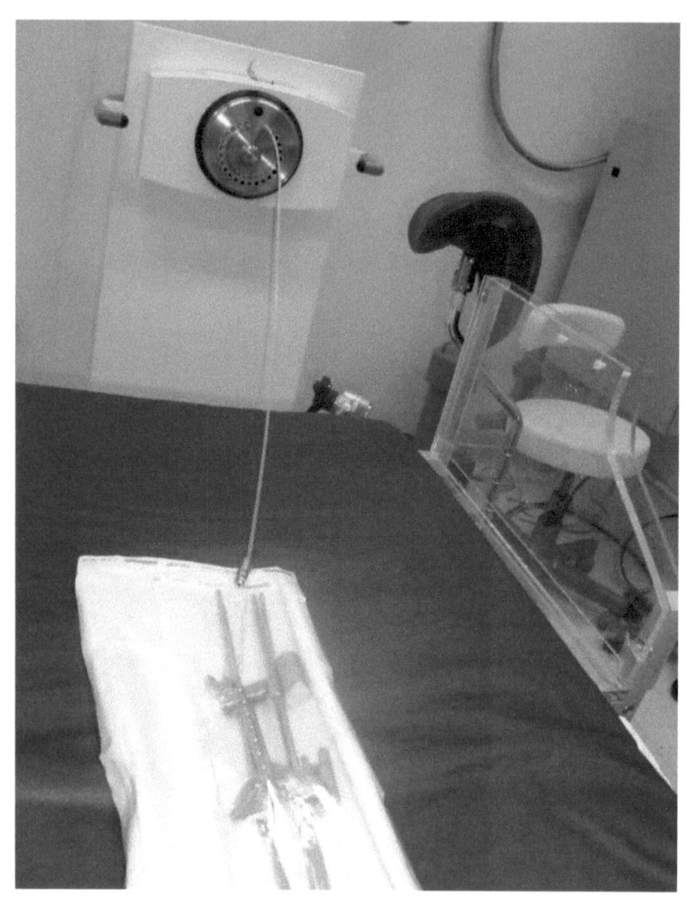

APPLICANTS

COLLECTION OF NURSE CLAUDIA ARAUJO

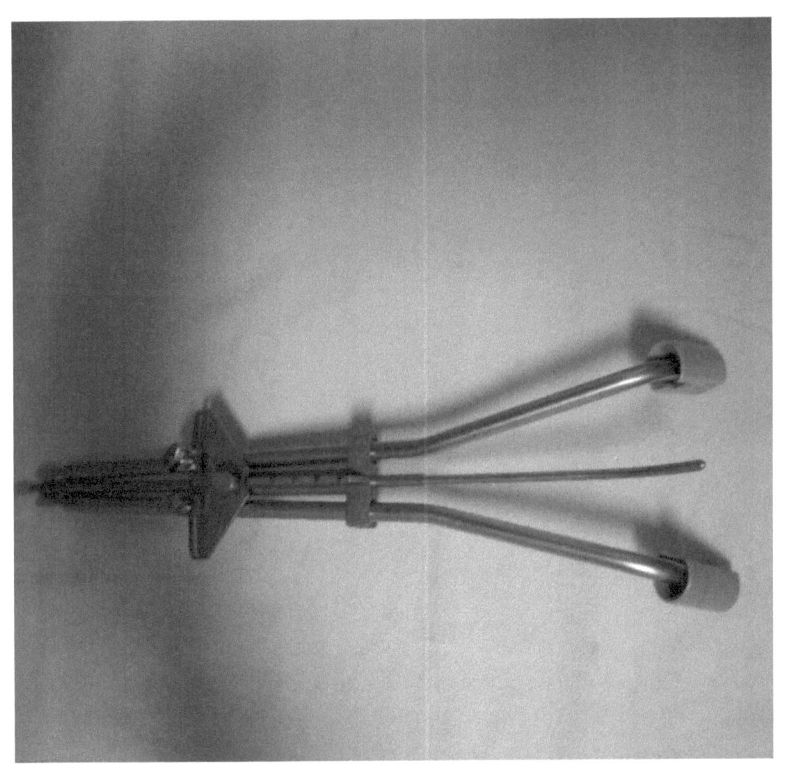

APPLICANTS

COLLECTION OF NURSE CLAUDIA ARAUJO

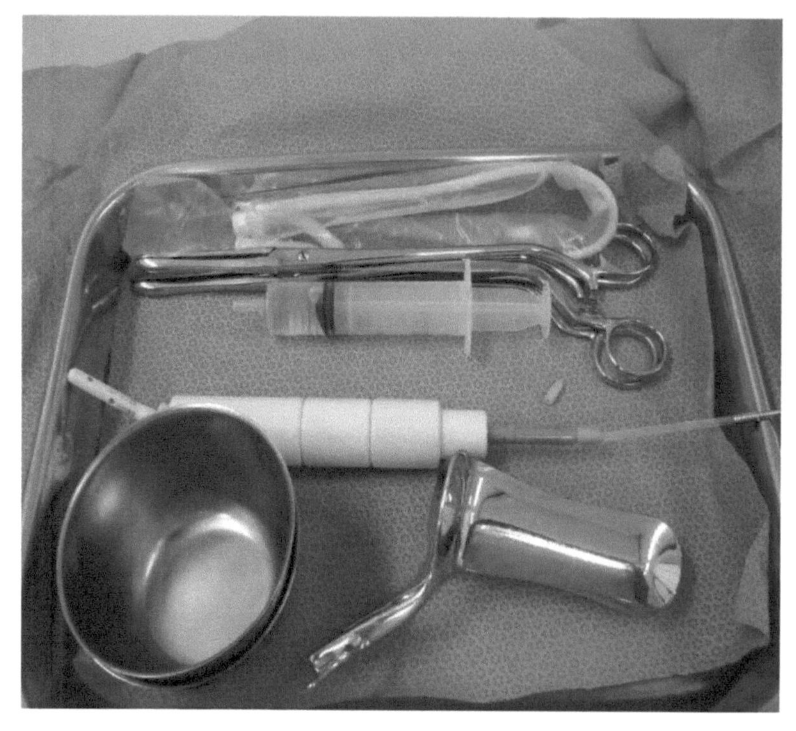

APPLICANTS

COLLECTION OF NURSE CLAUDIA ARAUJO

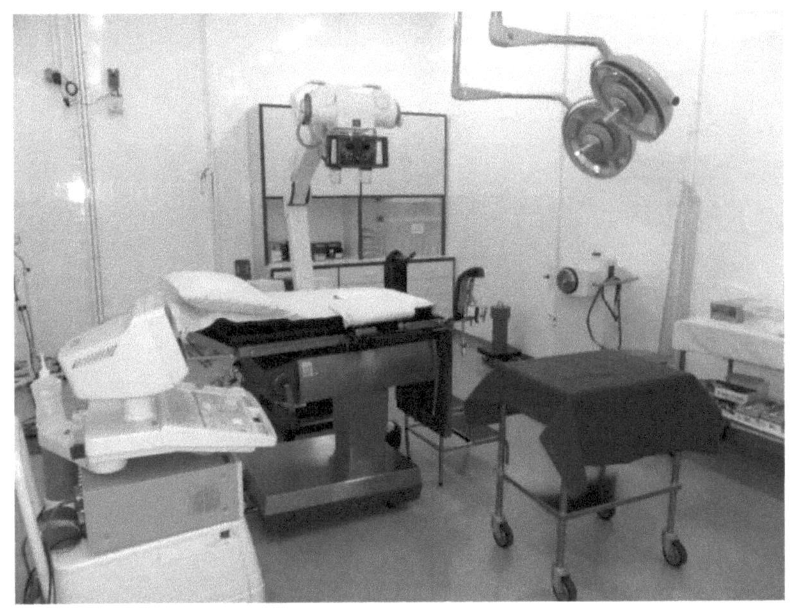

TREATMENT ROOM

COLLECTION OF THE NURSING TEAM AT THE PIO XII FOUNDATION'S BARRETOS CANCER HOSPITAL

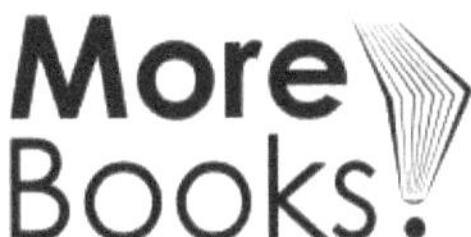

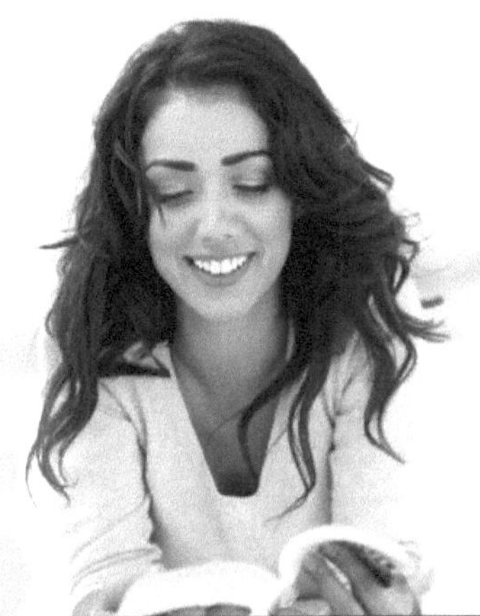

I want morebooks!

Buy your books fast and straightforward online - at one of world's fastest growing online book stores! Environmentally sound due to Print-on-Demand technologies.

Buy your books online at
www.morebooks.shop

Kaufen Sie Ihre Bücher schnell und unkompliziert online – auf einer der am schnellsten wachsenden Buchhandelsplattformen weltweit! Dank Print-On-Demand umwelt- und ressourcenschonend produziert.

Bücher schneller online kaufen
www.morebooks.shop

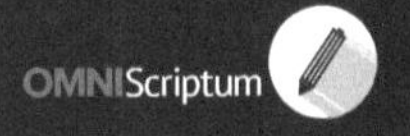

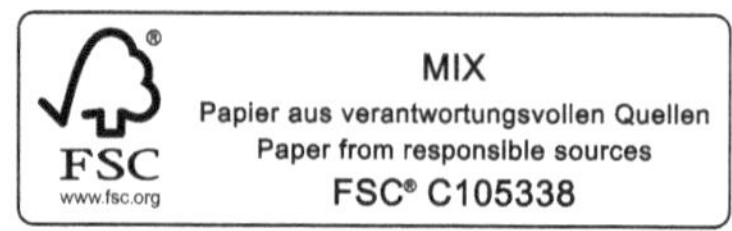

Printed by Books on Demand GmbH, Norderstedt / Germany